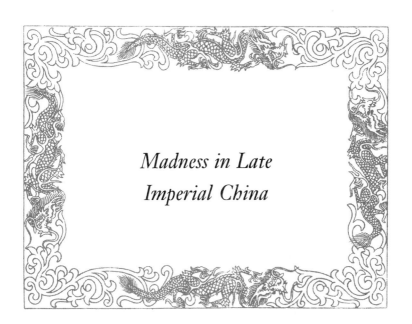

Madness in Late
Imperial China

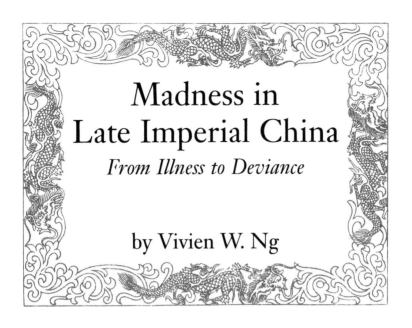

Madness in
Late Imperial China
From Illness to Deviance

by Vivien W. Ng

University of Oklahoma Press : Norman and London

This book is published with the aid of a grant from the Wallace C.
Thompson Endowment Fund, University of Oklahoma Foundation.

Library of Congress Cataloging-in-Publication Data
Ng, Vivien W. (Vivien Wai-ying)
    Madness in late imperial China : from illness to deviance / by
Vivien W. Ng.—1st ed.
        p.   cm.
    Includes bibliographical references and index.
    ISBN 0-8061-2297-8 (alk. paper)
    1. Mental illness—China—History.   2. Social psychiatry—
China—History.   3. China—History—Ch'ing dynasty,
1644–1916.   I. Title.
RC451.C6N666   1990
616.89′00951′0903—dc20   90-50237
                                                                CIP

The paper in this book meets the guidelines for permanence and
durability of the Committee on Production Guidelines for Book
Longevity of the Council on Library Resources, Inc. ∞

For Jenny

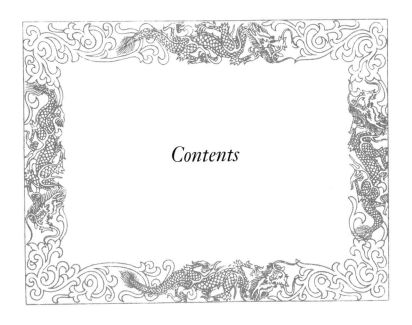

Contents

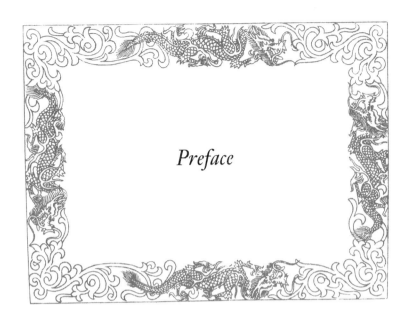

Preface

IN THE EIGHTEENTH CENTURY, for the first time in Chinese history, madness came to be perceived by law enforcement officials as a pressing problem. As a result, a number of unprecedented laws were enacted. These had two basic aims. First, to isolate the insane from the rest of society; and second, to recognize violent acts committed by the insane as serious crimes, and to make provisions for such crimes in the Qing legal code.

Madness was by no means a newly discovered medical problem. In fact, the Chinese had already amassed a wealth of knowledge regarding the subject. Madness was recognized as an illness as early as the first century A.D., when the compilation of the medical classic *Huangdi neijing* (Yellow Emperor's manual of corporeal medicine) was completed. Two major types of madness, *dian* and *kuang*, were discussed in this treatise. The *dian* condition was attributed to an overabundance of yin in a person's physiology, while *kuang* was believed to be caused by an excess of yang. As understanding of disease etiology became more sophisticated, explanations for the two maladies also became more complex. From the fourteenth century onward, references to the use of physical violence by insane persons (of the *kuang* type) appeared often in discourses on madness, but this awareness did not lead to any effort on the part of the Ming government to quarantine the insane.

The transformation of madness from an illness to a form of criminal deviance was not a result of new medical discoveries. What, then, was the impetus for such a dramatic change? A cursory look at the English and French experience offers an illuminating contrast, for during the nineteenth century, madness in these two societies was transformed from a form of deviance to an illness. What accounted for the change? Since scholars such as Andrew Scull and Michel Foucault have suggested that social and political change were major contributing factors in the European transformation, it is logical that we investigate the social and political climate of early Qing China to discern and identify possible reasons for change.

The decision to segregate the insane from the rest of Chinese society eventually led to the introduction of a mandatory registration-and-confinement program. This represented an intrusion of the government into family life, because families had to report to local officials the illness of their relatives and to take government-dictated steps to guarantee the safety of both the afflicted person and the community. How did Chinese families respond to this invasion? Did the government order make any sense to the general population? What obstacles were there to impede the implementation of such a draconian policy? The criminalization of madness also forced upon Qing jurists the burden of having to deal with the problem of criminal responsibility of the insane. How did Qing legal experts define insanity and/or insane behavior? What tests did they employ to determine insanity? Did physicians play any role in the evaluation of the state of mind of the criminal? In the absence of advocates for the accused, what guarantees were there to ensure fair treatment of insane offenders? Were Chinese criminals more disadvantaged than their counterparts in England, where the service of lawyers was available? Consideration of such questions helps us to understand not only the problem of insanity but Chinese cultural values as well.

The crux of this study is a charting of the legal aftermath of the transformation of madness from illness to deviance. This effort has been greatly facilitated by Xue Yunsheng's *Duli cunyi* (Commentary on Qing law) and Nakamura Shigeo's *Shindai keihō kenkyū* (Studies on Qing law). Xue Yunsheng, a late Qing legal scholar and one-time Board of Punishments official, commented extensively on most items in the Qing Code, and he often included the dates of enactment and revisions of many of the substatutes. Although some of his dates are not precise, his book is an indispensible source of information on enactment dates. Xue typically listed each substatute in its late-nineteenth-century form, followed by a notation regarding when the substatute was first enacted and subsequently revised. He did not, however, indicate which parts of a substatute were revisions. Fortunately, Nakamura Shigeo, through meticulous scholarship, has done precisely this for a large number of Qing laws concerning insane persons.

From primary sources I have culled over one hundred cases that contain specific references to the insane. The bulk of the cases came from the *Xing'an huilan* (Conspectus of penal cases) and *Xing'an huilan xupian* (Supplement to conspectus). Other sources include earlier collections, such as *Li'an chuanji* (Collection of legal precedents), *Cheng'an zhiyi* (Queries on leading cases) and *Cheng'an xinpian* (New collection of leading cases), as well as compilations published and distributed by the Board of Punishments, the Statutes Commission and provincial judicial offices. The primary purpose for the publication of these various compilations was to provide judicial officials with a ready source of reference for the disposition of cases, particularly unusual or problematic ones. Thus, only a very small percentage of the collections are what might be considered "open-and-shut" cases. Because of the nature of my sources, most of the cases presented in this book do not involve ordinary, commonplace situations. They are often complex and convoluted, but this is precisely their value. While following the sometimes tortuous routes taken by the Qing jurists in reaching a decision, we see diverse facets of the Qing judicial decision-making process and can observe the fascinating world of Qing law in action.

The sources that I have consulted for this research project, which include popular narrative literature as well as legal tracts, cases, and statutes, do not constitute an exhaustive collection of all extant materials on the subject of criminal insanity in Qing China. But, as John Carroll puts it, "Our task . . . is, like a still-photographer, to make detailed portraits of key moments, which, when viewed together, will bring about the lines of significant change" (1977, 11).

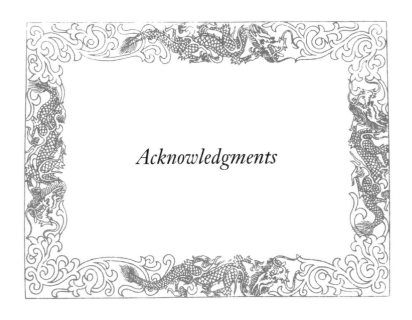

Acknowledgments

This study began as a graduate seminar paper and has under-gone numerous metamorphoses. Its present form is the culmi-nation of more than a decade of research and countless hours of fruitful discussion with friends, teachers, and colleagues. I would like to thank Professor Brian E. McKnight, my disser-tation advisor, for giving me free rein to unravel the puzzle of criminal insanity in Qing China at a time when I had only the vaguest notion of the depth and scope of the enterprise; Pro-fessor Harry J. Lamley for his guidance while I was writing the dissertation; Professor Jonathan D. Spence for his encourage-ment; Professor Richard J. Smith for his staunch support for this project; and the American Association of University

Women Educational Foundation for awarding me a doctoral research fellowship.

My most heartfelt thanks go to my friend Jennifer Robertson. She was there at the inception of the project and saw me through the exciting (but at times frustrating) research phase in Tokyo. I dedicate this book to her.

VIVIEN W. NG

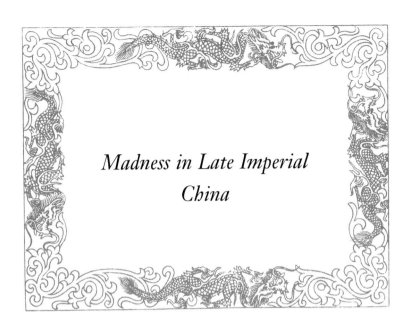

Madness in Late Imperial China

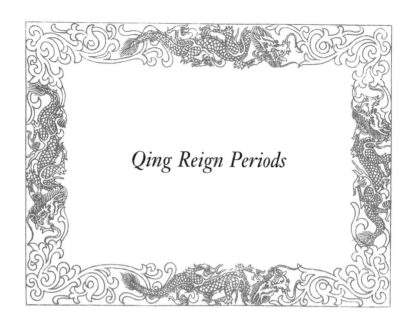

Qing Reign Periods

Reign Name	Years of Rule
Shunzhi	1644–1661
Kangxi	1662–1722
Yongzheng	1723–1735
Qianlong	1736–1795
Jiaqing	1796–1820
Daoguang	1821–1850
Xianfeng	1851–1850
Tongzhi	1862–1874
Guangxu	1875–1908
Xuantong	1909–1911

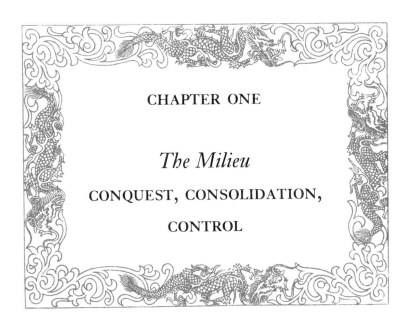

CHAPTER ONE

The Milieu

CONQUEST, CONSOLIDATION,

CONTROL

The Manchu Conquest

IN JUNE 1644, MANCHU TROOPS marched into the beleaguered Ming capital, Beijing. The new rulers of China found the inhabitants already confused and cowed by recent traumatic events. Some two months earlier the rebel Li Zicheng (the "dashing prince") laid seige on the city, forcing the Ming emperor Chongzhen to hang himself on Prospect Hill, overlooking the Forbidden City. The imperial suicide was soon followed by similar acts committed by some forty of his ministers, many of whom blamed themselves for the fall of the Ming dynasty. Within two days of the rebels' occupation of Beijing, commoners began to feel the pain of their undisciplined presence. Much of the looting (residents of Beijing called it "scouring") took place without Li's knowledge or permission, but his inability to curb the excesses of his lieutenants made him the focal point of the citizens' wrath (Wakeman 1985, chap. 4).

The total breakdown in political and social order inspired warlords into action. The role played by Wu Sangui during this critical juncture is the stuff of history as well as popular lore. Wu Sangui was commander of forty thousand regular Ming frontier troops posted at Ningyuan, just north of the Great Wall. In late April 1644, when the forces of Li Zicheng were advancing on Beijing, the Chongzhen emperor ordered Wu to send his men southward to the capital in order to help defend it. It soon became apparent that Wu was reluctant to do so, for he and his soldiers rode at a leisurely pace to Shanhaiguan (a key pass in the Great Wall) and then further south toward Beijing; in any case, the city fell before his arrival.

Most students of Chinese history are familiar with the ofttold tale about Wu's subsequent decision to enlist the help of the Manchus to rid Beijing of Li Zicheng. As the story goes, Wu was about to ally himself with the rebels when word got to him that his favorite concubine, Chen Yuan, had been seized and ravaged by Li Zicheng. Wu was so enraged that he decided on the spot not only to spurn Li's attractive offers but also to invite the Manchus into China to help him avenge his honor and slay the hated rebel leader (see, for example, Hsü 1970, 27). In fact, the circumstances that led to Wu's rejection of Li Zicheng were quite complicated and not as romantic as those presented in the popular account. Wu Sangui, however, did appeal to the Manchus for help. In May of 1644, when he knew that a protracted—and potentially disastrous—war with rebel troops was a certainty, he wrote a long and ingratiating letter to the newly enthroned Manchu emperor, Shunzhi, who was then only six years old. In the letter, Wu related the news that the Ming emperor had been overthrown by a "disorderly mob of petty thieves" (Wakeman 1985, 300). Chongzhen, he wrote, had been ill-served by his ministers: "The former emperor was unfortunate in that the loyalties of the capital's populace were not fixed, and a clique of traitors opened the gates and welcomed in the bandits" (ibid, 301). He would like to lead a righteous army against the rebels, but, regrettably, he lacked the resources to do so. Perhaps the Manchus could lend a hand? The rewards for them would be great, once the rebellion had been quelled. He promised them more territory north of the Great Wall to occupy, as well as a healthy share of the rebels' booty.

Wu Sangui's overture was the opportunity the Manchus had been waiting for. They had begun their quest for China some decades earlier under the brilliant leadership of Nurhaci (1559–1626), whose military successes at the turn of the seventeenth century had firmly established his hegemony over other tribal groups. In 1616, Nurhaci felt that he was ready to embark on the enterprise of empire-building. He announced the founding of a new dynasty (Jin) and bestowed on himself the title of khan (Mongolian for "emperor"). Although he did not live to see his dream realized, by the time of his death in 1626 he had annexed considerable territory along China's northeastern frontier and set his people on an irreversible collision course with the Ming state. In 1636, the Manchu khan Abahai (Nurhaci's eighth son and successor) took another bold symbolic step: he changed the dynastic title from Jin to Qing (pure), proclaimed himself emperor, and assumed the sinicized imperial name Taizong (see Wakeman 1985, chap. 1, 3). All that was left to accomplish was to overcome the stiff Chinese frontier defenses. Wu Sangui's offer to open the gates of Shanhaiguan for them was a godsend. It was thus that the Manchus crossed the Great Wall and marched all the way to Beijing, determined to stay.

The Manchus would have liked to settle into the task of governing China as peacefully as possible, but the use of military force was nonetheless necessary. The marauding bandit gangs, for example, had to be mopped up, and the stubborn Southern Ming court in Nanjing would not surrender without a fight. Even after the fall of the Southern Ming regime, Ming loyalists, particularly those living in South China—heartland of literati culture—continued to put up a stiff fight, forcing the Manchus to use brute force to break down their resistance. Even as they were contending with militant Ming loyalists, the Qing rulers also were putting down the rebellion of the Three

Feudatories (Wu Sangui in Yunnan and Guizhou, Shang Kexi in Guangdong, and Geng Jingzhong in Fujian). It was not until 1684, when the last stronghold of Ming loyalist resistance on Taiwan was quelled and the island officially incorporated into the province of Fujian, that Manchu rule over China was complete.

Extension of Imperial Control

Regent Dorgon knew at the outset that he had to take immediate steps to put the minds of the inhabitants of Beijing and surrounding communities at ease. Shortly after he entered the Ming capital in early June 1644, he issued several proclamations to the Chinese people, urging them not to be fearful. Mindful of the lootings committed by Li Zicheng's bandit gangs which had so antagonized the local populace, he ordered his officers to be careful not to disrupt the daily routine of the people (*Shizu shilu* 1937, 8:2a–3b; 7b–8a). To further assure the Chinese that the Manchu conquerors were not uncouth barbarians, Dorgon had collaborating Ming officials issue statements that advanced the image of the Manchus as civilized and well-behaved (Struve 1984, 58). In order to convince the Chinese that the Manchus were not transient raiders and to counter pernicious rumors of their imminent departure, Dorgon issued public announcements that the Qing regime was a permanent government (Wakeman 1985, 450–53). These assurances were a necessary part of his overall effort to usher in as quickly as possible an aura of stability and permanence to rebellion-torn China. The regent was also sensitive to the fact that years of disorder had badly unraveled the fabric of Chinese society. Both he and his key advisors were disturbed by the large number of litigations in newly pacified areas and correctly interpreted such contentiousness as a sign of social disintegration. Several times during the first year of the Shunzhi reign, people living in these areas were exhorted to desist from unnecessary litigation and to settle their disputes amicably (*Shizu shilu* 1937, *juan* 7, 8).

The new rulers of China faced the daunting task of reconstruction with vigor and determination, qualities that were sorely lacking in the Ming court during the decrepit final decades of the dynasty. In fact, late Ming ineptitude and corruption provided the Manchus a perfect foil for their reforms. The first order of business was to alleviate peasant distress, a priority that was dictated by pragmatic as well as humanitarian considerations. James Parsons has shown that the uprisings that wracked China in the first half of the seventeenth century had many causes, each having its own particular set of circumstances and conditions. Nonetheless, it is safe to say that the increasingly heavy tax burden imposed on the populace was a major contributing factor, one which was compounded in many instances by the poor performance of government officials (Parsons 1970).

The policies implemented by the nascent government to deal with the issues of official conduct and taxation were emblematic of Dorgon's determination to avoid repeating fatal mistakes made by the Ming. In late June 1644, the regent announced to the bureaucrats that he would not tolerate the "corrupt customs" of late Ming officialdom and that they should do their utmost to perform their duties well (Wakeman 1985, 448–49). He then proceeded quickly to lighten the tax burden of Chinese living in Manchu-controlled areas, cutting by about one-third their tax quota. In areas devastated by war and natural disaster, it was declared that taxes would be forgiven until economic recovery had taken place (Wakeman 1985, 450; Oxnam 1975, 41). Other reforms followed, all reflecting Dorgon's attempt to balance his authoritarian, no-nonsense approach to governance against an awareness of the demands of the Mandate of Heaven for benevolent rule. In fact, as Harold Kahn noted in his assessment of the personal styles of emperors Kangxi, Yongzheng, and Qianlong, authoritarianism and benevolence were hallmarks of the first 150 years of Qing rule:

> [Kangxi] (1662–1722) in his long reign consolidated the dynastic grip on the country, [Yongzheng] (1722–1736) tightened up the imperial control of administration, and [Qianlong] (1736–1795) profited from their success. The forte of all three was action, organization, and vigorous exercise of the imperial prerogatives. Perhaps more than previous dynasts, they recognized

the potentialities and made the most of their position. . . . At stake were the supremacy and majesty of the throne. The task was to exorcize the specter of destructive Ming factionalism, rationalize the Manchu overlordship, assert the primacy of the emperor. . . . Nevertheless it was not an obsession with power alone that controlled their view of the imperial vocation. The same Confucian tradition that provided the intellectual and ethical justification for their harsh and uncompromising views on leadership and loyalty also prescribed ideals of benevolence and humanity to which they would not be wholly indifferent. (Kahn 1971, 7–8)

Another characteristic of emperors Kangxi, Yongzheng, and Qianlong was their preference for tight personal control over the government. They inherited from Dorgon not only a strong centralized bureaucracy but a penchant for autocratic rule. Kangxi, for example, used bondservants as his agents to check on the bureaucracy and extend his grip on the empire (Spence 1966, 17). He also introduced a new system of communication between himself and individual officials. Under the traditional system, a typical memorial passed through many hands and several offices before it reached the emperor for decision and again before the final draft of the imperial rescript was delivered to the appropriate board for execution. Such a cumbersome system was at first deemed necessary because it prevented alteration of the emperor's final instructions. However, Silas Wu has pointed out that, "precisely because such a decision-making procedure involved so many people, secrecy was most difficult. Personal motives crept in, conflicts of interest arose, and tensions developed between the participants in the deliberative bodies and the emperor himself" (1970, 33). Finally, in the middle of his reign, Kangxi decided to implement a more streamlined procedure—the palace memorial system—which would provide him with ready access to raw information and allow quicker execution of imperial decisions. At the beginning, he invited only provincial officials to send secret memorials to him, but later, confronted with the knotty problem of imperial succession and the pernicious factional politics that attended it, he expanded the system to include court ministers. The following edict, issued in 1715, offered his rationale for the expanded system:

Rulers of past dynasties all discovered seditious and treacherous ministers. If the ruler detected their activities early, they could be quelled quietly, but if a ruler allowed such activities to spread, the harmful consequences became most serious later. It is indeed my own prescribed duty as emperor to labor day and night for the country and for the people but there are many things about which I have no means of obtaining information. Because of this, I have ordered the generals-in-chief, governors-general, commanders-in-chief, and brigade generals to enclose their secret memorials in their greetings palace memorials. Therefore all the affairs in the provinces cannot be concealed deceitfully. This practice has shown to be very beneficial and effective to the people's life and welfare. Since all of you are ministers whom I trust, you therefore ought to join the high provincial officials in presenting your reports on things which ought to be memorialized by enclosing them in your greetings palace memorials. . . .

If you [court ministers] could indeed report secretly according to the truth, then notoriously corrupt officials and notorious traitors would naturally become afraid of [being discovered], because they would not be able to know who has reported on them. These rascals who attempt to deceive their master [the emperor], and wield power illegally will naturally restrain themselves. I therefore have issued this special edict to you all! (ibid., 62–63)

Under Kangxi's successor, the emperor Yongzheng, the palace memorial system became more than a communication device employed by the emperor to collect raw and unadulterated information from the provinces and high-ranking officials. For the first time, palace memorials were used by a reigning emperor as "media for massive moral indoctrination and administrative rehabilitation of local officials" (ibid., 73). For example, in response to a palace memorial submitted by a governor-general, the emperor noted:

I have earnestly and repeatedly exhorted you and taught you. . . . If you could treat local affairs as if they were the business of your own family, and try to manage them tirelessly all the time, how could it be possible that you would not see any results? After three years, I want you to tell me that everything is all right. How could you expect me to trust what you have to say at the present time? After the three-year deadline is over, if I should find that your deeds are not in accordance with your words, you will certainly regret the consequences forever! Be very careful about this. (ibid., 74)

Even more overtly than was the case during the reign of Kangxi, the palace memorial was used as a device for mutual surveillance of officials. This was part of the "spy system" that Yongzheng installed to run his government; the palace memorial system was used by the emperor to assert more complete control over the bureaucracy in general (ibid., 76, 107).

The direct and autocratic character of early Qing rule was not just a consequence of imperial personality. "Lessons of the Ming" and the overall political milieu of the post-conquest period were major contributing factors as well. The Qing emperors did not have to go beyond the disastrous Wanli reign (1573–1620) of the late Ming dynasty to appreciate the dangers of indifferent rule (see Huang 1981 and Hegel 1981). Since one of the attributed causes for the Ming collapse was endemic (and systemic) official corruption, it was logical for the Manchu conquerors to adopt a more interventionist style to check the performance of officials and a more centralized system of government to facilitate such surveillance. Reform of the fiscal system during the early Qing period is a case in point. Madeleine Zelin explains it very well:

If the fiscal system established by the Ming founder was characterized by decentralization and the substitution of informal for formal mechanisms of control, the system that evolved during the early [Qing] was the opposite. The first generation of Chinese under Manchu rule witnessed the gradual development of a highly centralized system of tax administration and the evolution of a new, direct relationship between the taxpayer and the government.

As a first step, the [Qing] founders attempted to resolve

much of the chaos inherent in the Ming tax structure by placing
all taxes delineated in the [*Comprehensive Books of Taxation and
Services*] under the direct control of the central government. Instead of having each ministry of the central government collect
and manage its own revenues from the provinces, all central
government funds were now to be supervised by the Board of
Revenue. Moreover, under the first [Qing] emperor the Ming
proliferation of tax categories was eased and large numbers of
taxes were consolidated, with the result that the opportunities
for corruption and the confusion they entailed were eliminated.
(1984, 12–13)

The net result of early Qing fiscal reform was a strengthening
of the control of the central government over all the resources
of the empire (ibid., 26).

Ethnic minorities, too, were brought under direct central
control. Under the Ming, the tribal headmen system existed
more or less outside the pale of regular bureaucracy. Headmen
were chosen primarily from the chiefs of the non-Han groups;
although they were granted titles and ranks by the central government, they remained separate from regular bureaucrats
(Huang 1974, 281). When the Three Feudatories rebelled
against the Qing, their leaders recruited support from the
tribal chiefs of the non-Han groups, most notably the Miao,
Yao, and Lolo. After the rebellion was quelled, the Qing government initiated a thorough review of the tribal headmen
system, for the purpose of preventing similar subversive activities. One result was, as Pei Huang puts it, "the bureaucratiza-
tion" of the system. Several tribal regions were brought under
direct bureaucratic control. In Guizhou, for example, where
one could find a total of ninety-four different tribal units, six-
teen were incorporated into the regular administrative structure during the years 1684–1720 (ibid., 285). During the
Yongzheng reign, an even more aggressive policy was pursued.
One by one, tribal headmen were replaced by regular bureaucrats. Pei Huang sums up the process very well: "The development of southwest China, which originated mainly in the
[Yongzheng] Emperor's new ethnic minority policy, contrib-

uted to the extension of the imperial authority and consolidation of the southwestern interior frontiers of China" (ibid., 301).

The tenacity of Ming loyalist resistance, the rebellion of the Three Feudatories, and the legacy of the debilitating decades of peasant unrest all contributed to the early Qing obsession with law and order as well as its intolerance of nonconformity. The Qing rulers used both persuasion and coercion in their persistent effort to create a stable society made up of law-abiding conformists. No social class was able to escape the intrusion of the government into private life.

Regulation of Chinese Society

Mindful of the fact that the vast majority of the Chinese population were peasants who could not read printed didactic texts, the government revived an old method of popular instruction, *xiangyue*, the "village lecture system." Twice a month, on the first and fifteenth days, an appointed lecturer and his assistant would expound on the values considered most desirable by the Qing regime to a gathering composed of local elders, scholars, and commoners (Hsiao 1960, 185–86; Mair 1985, 350–51). In order to reinforce the message of the lectures, the names of persons guilty of social misconduct—for example, unfilial behavior—were posted in special kiosks. These names were removed only after it had been determined that the offenders had reformed their deviant ways (Hsiao 1960, 185–86). Another means of popular indoctrination resurrected by the Qing government was the so-called "community drinking ceremony." This compulsory affair was held twice a year at the district or prefectural seat and attended by members of the local gentry as well as a few select village elders. The sole purpose of the ceremony was to provide Qing authorities with another opportunity to explicate the importance of state-approved virtues such as respect for the aged, filial piety, chastity, loyalty, fraternity, and good neighborliness (ibid., 208). These, of course, were values cherished by conservative Chinese scholars, whose loyalty the Qing tried very hard to cultivate. The need to win over such scholars, however, did not eclipse the equally compelling need to control them.

Because the literati were so important to the state, they had to be kept in check, and the government spared no effort to limit the scope of their intellectual freedom as soon as it could afford to do so. Aware of the activist tradition of private academies, the early Qing rulers initially made some tentative attempts to stem their proliferation. However, they soon realized that a better alternative was to appropriate for their own use the academy system as a tool for ideological control. In 1733, for example, the Yongzheng emperor ordered the establishment of twenty-one government-subsidized "private" academies throughout the empire. To improve their competitive edge over the truly private institutions, students attending these schools, as well as their teachers, received stipends from the government. Later the same year, the emperor inaugurated imperial supervision over all academies. Eight years later, in an effort to standardize and control the content of local education, the government provided all schools with approved textbooks (Hsiao 1960, 235–36; Huang 1974, 203–204).

Ideological control of the literati was not limited to molding the minds of future generations of intellectuals; it also included suppressing unorthodox literary efforts of mature scholars. The literary inquisitions of the Kangxi, Yongzheng, and Qianlong periods served notice to the literati that nonconformist writings would not be tolerated by the government. During the Yongzheng period, for example, "inspectors of morale" were appointed by the emperor to keep an eye on the activities of both budding and mature scholars, and to supervise educational and examination programs. They were also responsible for keeping under strict surveillance those scholars who had been convicted of writing heterodox works. Under the Qianlong emperor, literary inquisition went beyond mere author suppression to become a large-scale, systematic effort to search out and destroy all "seditious" works (Hsiao 1960, 241; Goodrich 1966, 30–42; Guy 1987, 26–34).

Besides popular indoctrination and suppression of heterodox writings, imperial control included surveillance of the day-to-day activities of the populace. The ancient *baojia* or "mutual responsibility" system was reinstated partly for the purpose of police control. Under this system, each household was required to post a door placard on which were written the names of its members. This method of registration was obviously intended to allow surveillance personnel quickly to learn of strangers in the community. Households were grouped in units of ten: ten households were arranged into a *pai;* ten *pai* constituted a *jia;* ten *jia* formed a *bao.* In the edict of 1708 that revived this system, it was made clear that the principle of group responsibility would be applied (Sprenkel 1977, 47). Each registered person was required to report to his unit head any crimes committed in his neighborhood as well as the presence of any suspicious persons. The unit head, in turn, was required to relay such information to the next responsible person. Just as each household was responsible for the behavior of individual members, each unit was made accountable for the conduct of member households (Hsiao 1960, 28, 44–45). Another instrument of control, particularly in the rural areas, was the office of *dibao* (local constabulary). The *dibao* was directly responsible to the district magistrate and served as an important intermediary between the magistrate and the common people. His duties included passing on to his fellow villagers directives and demands of the magistrate and he was held personally responsible for their compliance. He also had a role to play in popular indoctrination: on the first and fifteenth days of each month, he read out the Sacred Edict of the emperor to his compatriots (Sprenkel 1977, 47). In localities where the *baojia* system was not functioning properly, the office of *dibao* filled the vacuum by assuming the responsibilities of the *baojia* and thus became the premier instrument of rural control (Sweeten 1976, 4–5). The *baojia* and *dibao* systems later emerged as key components in the Qing response to the problem of insanity (see Chapter Three).

Very early on, the Qing government recognized in the law codes a potent tool for social engineering. One example of this awareness is the rape statute of 1646 which imposed very stringent evidential requirements for rape charges. The intent of this law was to promote the cult of female chastity (see Ng 1987). Using law (*fa*) to promote morality (*li*) was not a Qing innovation; rather it was a tradition of very long standing, dating all the way back to the early Han period, when a merging of Confucian idealism with Legalist pragmatism was effected. Prior to the Han synthesis, Confucianism and Legalism were two irreconcilable schools of thought, especially with respect to their theories concerning the use of law and punishment. Confucius himself was unequivocal in his insistence that a ruler should use moral suasion, rather than coercion, to govern his people. In the *Analects*, for example, he said, "Lead the people with governmental measures and regulate them by law and punishment, and they will avoid wrong doing but will have no sense of honor and shame. Lead them with virtue and regulate them by the rules of propriety (*li*), and they will have a sense of shame and, moreover, set themselves right" (Chan 1973, 22). In stark contrast, Legalists insisted that the proper function of a ruler was not to serve his people but to create and maintain a strong state. Toward this end, he must rely on the rule of law and not be afraid to employ harsh punishments.

Confucianism triumphed over Legalism with the establishment of the Han dynasty, when it was adopted as the orthodox ideology. The statesman who played an instrumental role in making Confucianism the state doctrine of Han China was Dong Zhongshu (c. 179–104 B.C.). His contribution to the unfolding of Han Confucian thought can be found in two other areas: the introduction of the concept of *sangang*—the Three Bonds between ruler and subject, father and son, husband and wife—and his elaboration of the theory of cosmic harmony. These two concepts eventually became key components of Chinese legal thought and judicial procedure.

Once charged with the responsibility of governing a vast empire, Han Confucianists realized that moral suasion alone could not maintain a stable society and that a heavy dose of Legalist pragmatism was necessary. What ensued was a gradual process of synthesis: in the area of law, this process has been characterized by legal historians as "Confucianization of law." If law must be employed by the state, then it should be used to promote Confucian values as well as to maintain order in society. Laws enacted by successive dynasties to bolster the hierarchical structure of the family offer an excellent example of the relation of law to morality in Confucian China. The family was the center of the Chinese social and moral universe. Two of the hallowed Three Bonds, for example, defined familial relations (father-son, husband-wife). Ideally, members of a family were linked to one another by a web of ethical ties, and the roles and responsibilities of each member were defined by the individual's position within the family. Status was determined by three factors: generation, age, and sex. In the words of Richard J. Smith, "The theme of Chinese family life (and social life generally) was subordination: the individual to the group, the [young] to the [old], and females to males" (1983, 65). Status privileges and obligations were dictated by a system of intrafamily relations called *wufu*, "five mourning degrees." It is important to note that in all degrees of mourning, "the linkage is through the male line, so that 'cousin' means only a father's brother's son, not a father's sister's son or daughter" (ibid., 67). This system also found application in Chinese law, and successive dynasties used it as a guide for determining appropriate punishment for crimes committed by one family member against another.

The Manchu government embraced wholeheartedly the Confucian vision of the family. Until nearly the end of the Qing dynasty, when attempts were made to modernize Chinese law, senior members of a family or clan enjoyed a number of legal privileges, often at the expense of their juniors. Like earlier dynasts, Qing rulers found Confucian family values such as filial piety, respect for the aged, and female chastity compatible with their efforts to create and maintain a stable and authority-abiding society. The emperor Yongzheng was especially vigorous in his promotion of filial piety. Shortly after his succession to the throne he restored the *Xiaojing* (Canon of filial piety) to the list of books required for civil service examinations; a few years later he ordered its publication in both Chinese and Manchu. In fact, he promoted it with

Table 1. The Five Degrees of Mourning

Degree	Appropriate apparel	Duration of mourning	Relationships requiring specific degree of mourning
1 *Zhancui*	Unhemmed sackcloth	3 years	Mourning by a man for his parents By a woman for her husband or husband's parents
2 *Zicui*	Hemmed sackcloth	1 year (or less)	By a man for his grandparents, uncle, uncle's wife, spinster aunt, brother, spinster sister, wife, son, daughter-in-law (wife of first-born), nephew, spinster niece, or grandson (first-born son of first-born) By a woman for her husband's nephew, husband's spinster niece, parents, or grandparents
3 *Dagong*	Coarse cotton	9 months	By a man for his married aunt, married sister, brother's wife, first cousin, daughter-in-law (wife of a younger son), nephew's wife, married niece, or grandson By a woman for her husband's grandparents, husband's uncle, husband's daughter-in-law, husband's nephew's wife, husband's nephew's wife, husband's married niece, or grandson
4 *Xiaogong*	Less coarse cotton than for *dagong*	5 months	By a man for his granduncle, granduncle's wife, etc.
5 *Sima*	Plain hempen cloth	3 months	By a man for his great granduncle, great granduncle's wife, spinster great grandaunt, etc.

Source: Adapted from Smith (1983), 66–67.

such zeal that, in the words of Pei Huang, "the *Canon of Filial Piety* became increasingly a political instrument for his autocratic purposes" (1974, 197). Following a tradition that dated back to the Han period, the Qing listed parricide and "lack of filial piety" as two of ten unpardonable offenses or "abominations." The Qing Code also provided that a son who dared to strike his parent suffered decapitation, regardless of whether injury was inflicted (Bodde and Morris 1973, 37). The provision in dynastic codes of severe punishments for offenses that violate cardinal Confucian values shows that "Confucianization of law" meant not only the use of law to promote morality but also acceptance of the Legalist position of using punishment to discourage and penalize deviant behavior. The Qing regime did not hesitate to use the legal code to proscribe "aberrant" conduct. For example, in 1740, the government enacted its first male homosexual rape law. However, this law addressed more than the issue of rape because buried in this substatute is the criminalization of male homosexuality, with sodomy between consenting adults a punishable offense. This homophobic legislation had a number of contributing causes, one of which was the political climate of the early Qing period. John Boswell's study of homosexuality in Europe reveals striking parallels with the Qing. According to Boswell, the onset of homophobia in Europe in the late Middle Ages coincided with the rise of absolute government. It is clear that political developments played a large role in the narrowing of social tolerance in Europe. Boswell noted a push for intellectual and institutional uniformity: "Theology was fitted in systematic formulas and collected in comprehensive compendia— summas of such formulas. The Inquisition arose to eliminate theological loose ends and divergence of opinion. Secular knowledge was gathered into uniform approaches, encyclopedia, which attempted to unite all of contemporary learning into one book or system" (1980: 270). Substitute philosophical orthodoxy for theology, and we have an apt description of early Qing intellectual and political developments. It is possible that the government regarded homosexuality as the ultimate form of heterodox, iconoclastic expression and, therefore, took steps to outlaw it. It is also possible that conservative elements within the government viewed homosexuals as gender anomalies and, as such, portents of a state of cosmic imbalance or disharmony that required rectification.

The theory of cosmic correspondences and harmony evolved in China during the Warring States period, a time of tremendous philosophical development, but it was Dong Zhongshu, the celebrated Han scholar, who gave the theory its most elaborate form. In his treatise *Chunqiu fanlu* (Luxuriant gems of the *Spring and autumn annals*), Dong made the following observation:

> A beautiful thing calls forth things that are beautiful in kind and an ugly thing calls forth things that are ugly in kind, for things of the same kind arise in response to each other. For example, when a horse neighs, it is horses that will respond, [and when an ox lows, it is oxen that will respond]. Similarly, when an emperor or king is about to rise, auspicious omens will first appear, and when is he about to perish, unlucky omens will first appear. . . .
>
> Heaven possesses yin and yang and man also possesses yin and yang. When the universe's material force of yin arises, man's material force of yin arises in response. Conversely, when man's material force of yin arises, that of the universe should also arise in response. The principle is the same. He who understands this, when he wishes to bring forth rain, will activate the yin in man in order to arouse the yin of the universe. . . . Even the way misfortunes, calamities, and blessings are produced follows the same principle. In all cases one starts something himself and other things become active in response according to their kind. (Chan 1973, 283–84)

As Wing-tsit Chan noted in his discussion of this treatise, "the belief in portents is as old as Chinese thought. What is new in [Dong Zhongshu] is that he explains it in terms of natural law. Instead of expressions of the pleasure or displeasure of spiritual beings, portents are results of the cosmic material forces of yin and yang" (ibid., 283).

The theory of cosmic harmony became an integral part of Han Confucianism. Subsequently, the process of Confucian-Legalist synthesis effected the "naturalization" of law, leading eventually to the subordination of law to the movements of nature (Bodde and Morris 1973, 44). Thus, from the Han dynasty on, it was not uncommon for an emperor to declare an amnesty in response to a series of natural catastrophes. In A.D. 28, for example, Emperor Guangwu issued this edict:

A long-time drought is harmful to the wheat crops. Now the autumn seed has not yet been put into the soil. We are worrying about it. Is this due to the fact that cruel officials are still in action, that most of the judicial cases are unfairly settled, and that the sadness and grievances of the people have impressed Heaven? Let all the prisoners in the capital and in the various provinces be released; let those who are not subject to death sentences not be examined; and let those who are now imprisoned be freed and become common people. (Ch'ü 1961, 214)

The notion that miscarriage of justice might lead to natural calamities dictated the need to regulate against possible abuses by judicial officials. During the Qing period, for example, judges were required to cite relevant statutes or substatutes in rendering their decisions. Fu-mei Chang Chen's research has led her to conclude that "the government seems to have been most successful in enforcing these requirements through a rigid review system" (1970, 213). The government also instituted at least five levels of review for capital offenses. The emperor was the final arbiter in all capital cases, a responsibility that seemed to have caused Kangxi considerable anguish:

Giving life to people and killing people—those are the powers that the emperor has. He knows that administrative errors in government bureaus can be rectified, but that a criminal who has been executed cannot be brought back to life any more than a chopped string can be joined together again. He knows, too, that sometimes people have to be persuaded into morality by the example of an execution. In 1683, after Taiwan had been captured, the court lecturers and I discussed the image of the fifty-sixth hexagram in the *Book of Changes*, "Fire on the Mountain": the calm of the mountain signifies the care that must be used in imposing penalties; the fire moves rapidly on, burning up the grass, like lawsuits that should be settled speedily. My reading of this was that the ruler needs both clarity and care in punishing: his intent must be to punish in order to avoid the need for further punishing. . . .

But apart from . . . treason cases, when there are men who have to be executed immediately (even if it's spring, when executions should not be carried out), or when one is dealing with men like those who plotted against me in the Heir-Apparent crisis and had to be killed immediately and secretly without trial, I have been merciful where possible. For the ruler must always check carefully before executions, and leave room for the hope that men will get better if they are given the time. In the hunt one can kill all the animals caught inside the circle, but one can't always bear to shoot them as they stand there, trapped and exhausted. (Spence 1974, 29–31)

The other side of the concern for cosmic harmony is that in order to right wrongs, punishment appropriate to the nature of the offense must be meted out. This need was the most common reason for the use of analogy in Qing law. In the words of Fu-mei Chang Chen, "The use of analogy almost always involves [the] search for 'the most fitting punishment' for an unquestionably criminal act. This was necessary because [Qing] statutes, unlike most Western criminal laws, did not confer upon judges a broad discretionary power in sentencing" (1970, 216).

A few months into their occupation of China, the new rulers began reviewing the Ming Code for possible adoption by the Qing. This process proved to be a protracted one, a situation that Board of Punishments official Yang Huang found very disturbing. In 1646—the third year of Shunzhi's reign—Yang submitted a memorial to the emperor registering his concern that in the absence of a dynastic code, the people lacked a reference by which they could lead their lives. Not only did criminal offenders not know the reasons for their culpability, but enforcers of the law had been prone to mete out arbitrary sentences. He believed that China was in a state of legal anomie, and called for the speedy issuance of the official Qing Code (*Shizu shilu* 1937, 26:21a).

The Qing finally issued its first code in 1646 using the Ming Code as its model. The primary framework of the Qing Code was made up of more than four hundred *lü* (statutes), the bulk of which were inherited, with some modifications, from the Ming Code. The statutes were supplemented by a body of laws called *li* (substatutes), which provided much-needed flexibility to the legal system. Thomas Metzger makes the following observation:

Law or rule making, the making and excising of precedents and laws, was a continuous and basic process of the [Qing] state. . . . The frequency and importance of [Qing] law making are one illustration of the [Qing] state's flexibility. Probably flexibility can be found in any organization, however "tradition-bound," and some rigidity or fixation on ideals located in the past can be found in even the most modern organization. Therefore, variations between organizations in terms of flexibility should perhaps be seen as variations in the mix between tendencies to flexibility and rigidity. Yet sinologists have often been content to view the imperial Chinese state as dominated by an "atmosphere of routine, traditionalism, and immobility" without asking how the latter atmosphere was mixed with the tendencies toward flexibility. There has even been a tendency to think of the [Qing] state as simply "rigid." While the bureaucrats lazily sat on their power, we are sometimes told, people of all ranks busily and dynamically went about violating the laws. What is sometimes overlooked is that the laws would not have been enforced even to the extent that they were, were it not that the bureaucrats also were busy, continuously and flexibly making adjustments in response to the tendencies toward deviancy. It is this busy activity on both sides—the legal and the illegal—which constituted the life of [Qing] bureaucracy. (1973, 21–22)

If the Qing penal code had been made up of *lü* only, the legal system might not have been able to cope with social change. Metzger discerned a noticeable reluctance on the part of many Qing officials and even legal scholars to countenance the suggestion that *lü* could be altered. Indeed, "Confucianization of law" had resulted in the elevation of codified law to sanctified status. Even though the Qing regime did in fact alter a number of Ming *lü* in the 1646 edition of the Qing Code and made further changes in subsequent editions, Qing legal scholars generally preferred, as Metzger put it, to "gloss over" these changes, so eager were they to stress the continuity between the Qing and earlier periods (ibid., 84–85).

However, the Qing penal code was not made up of statutes only; it included also a supplemental body of laws—the substatutes (*li*)—which gave flexibility to the legal system. Substatutes were a Ming innovation which allowed change within tradition. A substatute usually originated as an imperial edict issued to deal with a particular situation, or as a precedent-setting judgment by the Board of Punishments concerning a case whose peculiar circumstances were not covered by an existing law. The edict or precedent was supposed to be binding on future decisions, but until it was recommended by the Statutes Commission for incorporation into the Qing Code as a substatute, many judicial officials appeared uncertain about its applicability. Once a decision became a substatute, it had primacy over the umbrella statute if there was a conflict between the two.

When the first Qing Code was issued in 1646, it contained only 449 substatutes. By 1863, the number had reached the peak figure of 1,892 (Chen 1970, 215). Some of these later substatutes were responses to new problems. For example, when opium smoking, a minor transgression in the seventeenth century, became a serious social problem in the eighteenth and nineteenth centuries, it triggered a volley of legislative activities aimed at combating both the cultivation and consumption of opium (Spence 1975, 143–73). Frequently, the substatutes themselves were amended, and each amendment was necessitated by the need to tackle conditions or situations which were not accommodated or anticipated by the original substatute. Fu-mei Chang Chen is of the opinion that in spite of the proliferation of substatutes during the Qing period, there were very few new crimes. This means that the substatute enactment process was more one of refinement than innovation (Chen 1970, 215). Seen in this light, the substatutes enacted by the Qing government to deal with criminal insanity acquire an even more exceptional meaning.

The village lectures, community drinking ceremonies, government-subsidized schools, literary inquisitions, *baojia* and *dibao* systems, and the Qing Code were employed by the state as instruments of social control. However, in spite of persistent efforts to regulate all aspects of life, the autocratic government's hold over society was in fact far from absolute. One of the political ironies of late imperial China is that the very institution the government worked hard to support was at the same time its greatest potential enemy. Forced to choose between the interests of the family and those of the state, most Chinese would opt for the former. Therefore, government policies which could undermine the integrity of the family stood very little chance of compliance. This reality had tremendous impact on the effectiveness of the Qing response to the problem of criminal insanity.

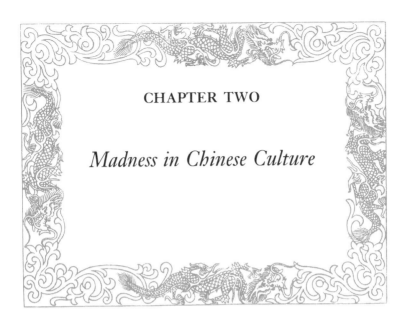

CHAPTER TWO

Madness in Chinese Culture

In 1702, FATHER JEAN-FRANÇOIS FOUQUET, a Jesuit assigned to the Catholic mission in Jiangxi province, wrote to a friend in France a letter detailing a very peculiar incident. In a village neighboring the town of Fuzhou, there lived a young woman who was afflicted with episodic fits of madness. Most of the time, she behaved in a normal fashion; periodically, however, she lost touch with reality. She would then describe her hallucinations very vividly, and often it was difficult for others to tell whether she was depicting an actual event or a figment of her delusion.

A number of Catholic cathecists were active in the region, and when they caught wind of her affliction, they approached her and preached to her the fundamentals of the Catholic faith. Their efforts had some effect on her, but unfortunately not in the way they had intended. She began making the sign of the cross and fussing with holy water, and when her curious neighbors asked her why she acted in such a manner, all she would say was that both the cross and holy water were "as fearful as death itself."

Her worried family consulted a number of physicians and different kinds of medicine were tried but nothing seemed to work. Just when the family was about to give up hope, a Daoist master, who called himself Zhang Tianshi (Heavenly Master Zhang), happened to pay a visit to Fuzhou. Zhang urged all the residents of the town to come to him with their troubles and ailments, for he had the means to alleviate them. Consequently, Fouquet wrote, "All the sick and unfortunate people of Fuzhou flocked to the Tianshi, hoping that he would deliver them from their troubles."

Driven by desperation, the young woman's family also sought help from the Tianshi and his entourage. They purchased a religious charm and other paraphernalia from the Daoists, hoping that such items would rid their beloved relative of her dreadful affliction. However, the woman's condition remained unchanged. Her family did not immediately give up hope; instead, they returned to the Daoists for more help, three times in all.

On each occasion, according to Fouquet, the Daoist "swindlers" slit the throats of a rooster, a dog, and a pig and offered the animals as a sacrifice. Fouquet reported that these rites proved to be entirely useless, but he noted sarcastically that the Daoists did enjoy feasting on the sacrificial animals. After the third failed attempt, the young woman was taken back to her natal home, for it was hoped that a change of abode would change her fortune. Unfortunately, not only did the move fail to solve the problem, but her illness soon became "contagious"—four of her young male relatives also began to act very strangely and, at times, violently.

Finally, a Catholic friend of the family suggested that their problem was caused by the devil and recommended formal conversion to Catholicism as their only recourse. The family, "desperately in need of help from God," sent someone to a Jesuit priest named Chavagnac to ask him for help. At first, Father Chavagnac refused to have anything to do with them because he thought that they were too deeply rooted in idolatry for him to be of any help. When the family learned of the priest's reservations, they removed all the "vestiges of paganism" from their house and turned them over to him, so that he would be convinced of their sincere intentions. Chavagnac finally relented. He selected a few of his trusted disciples and sent them to the young woman's home with precise instructions. Fouquet detailed the subsequent development in his letter:

> Armed with a crucifix, a small figurine of Jesus, rosaries, and holy water, the disciples made their way to the sick people's house. Immediately upon their arrival, the fits of madness dissipated and vanished. A Buddhist priest who witnessed this miracle, instead of giving praise to the Lord, dismissed the cure as mere happenstance. But the Almighty God, in order to demonstrate once and for all that the illness was cured by the disciples, allowed the symptoms of madness to reappear. Under the watchful eyes of everyone present, the disciples attended to the five supplicants. They hung rosaries on the necks of some and poured holy water on the others. Once again, the raving madness subsided. The disciples then placed a crucifix at the most prominent place in the house; vessels of holy water and some candles were also set down in various parts of the house.
>
> Needless to say, the cure was complete and permanent. From this time on the family was spared the ruckus and commotion that frequently accompanied the fits of madness.

In the wake of the "miracle," eight members of the young woman's family declared their intentions to become Christians. At the insistence of the pastor, they received catechism before they were baptized. Ironically, the young woman, whose recovery was the cause of this sudden display of devotion, steadfastly resisted all attempts to convert her. A disappointed Father Fouquet noted ruefully that "God's will simply cannot be fathomed" (Yazawa 1970, 22–26).

The eclectic, idiosyncratic, yet pragmatic response of the

young woman's family to her illness was typically Chinese. As Emily Ahern points out, the choice of healer depends largely on the patient's (or the family's) perception of the cause of an illness (1978, 101–10). At the onset of the illness of the young woman in Fuzhou, the family perceived her madness as organic in nature, thus they turned to physicians and herbal medicines for cure. But when her condition failed to improve, they conjectured that they had been mistaken and attributed her illness to supernatural causes, and so they appealed first to Daoists and later to Catholics for help.

There were two levels of traditional explanations and cures for madness. One level consisted of explanations expressed in "natural" terms such as yinyang, five evolutive phases, and emotions. Such explanations, found primarily in medical texts, reflected the views of the elite. The other level consisted of explanations expressed in "supernatural" terms such as spirit-possession, loss of the soul, and divine retribution. Such explanations, found primarily in stories, folk wisdom and folklore, typically reflected the views of the common people. These two levels of explanations, however, were not mutually exclusive.

Theoretical Foundations of Classical Chinese Medicine

Qing physicians were heirs to a long and rich medical tradition. The theoretical foundations of classical Chinese medicine were already firmly laid by first century A.D., and these were well articulated in the classic *Huangdi neijing* (Yellow Emperor's manual of corporeal medicine), the oldest extant Chinese medical text. Through the ages, more sophisticated and complex understanding of disease etiology continued to be added to this basic theoretical core, thus classical Chinese medicine by the Qing period was the sum total of almost two thousand years of evolution.

Precise dating of ancient Chinese medical texts is, at best, a problematic task. As M. Porkert points out, the transmission of the ancient texts is "submerged in utter darkness from the end of the Han well into the Sui period" (1974, 4). A case in point is *Huangdi neijing*. It is impossible to accurately place the exact date of its compilation. Textual analyses reveal sections that clearly are products of different epochs. Also, we now know that with the passage of time, many parts of the work were lost. Some of the lacunae were filled by the Tang commentator Wang Bing, who claimed to have consulted other ancient texts. It is highly probable, however, that Wang fabricated the restored sections himself (Jia 1979, 47–48). The best scholars have managed to determine is that the *Huangdi neijing* probably was a composite of many different medical treatises, some of them dating back to the Warring States period (fifth to third century B.C.), and that the compilation was more or less completed sometime during first century A.D. (Jia 1979, 48). In spite of its antiquity, the *Huangdi neijing*, in its usual two-part format (*Suwen* and *Lingshu*), remains today the most basic Chinese medical text.

The most fundamental component of classical Chinese medical theory, the yinyang system of correspondences, was well developed in the *Huangdi neijing*. Joseph Needham defines yin and yang as "fundamental forces" (1956, 273). In his exhaustive study of the theoretical foundations of Chinese medicine, Porkert defines yang as the "active aspect of an effective position," and yin as the "structive aspect of an effective position" (1974, 14). He further presents the following comparative summary of the fundamental associations of yin and yang: Yin corresponds to all that is structive, contractive, intrasusceptive (absorbing into or within the individual), centripetal, responsive, conservative, and positive. Yang, on the other hand, corresponds to all that is active, expansive, extraversive (bringing to the surface), centrifugal, aggressive, demanding, and negative (ibid., 23).

The yinyang system of correspondences is a dynamic one. Margaret Lock explains it as follows:

> The subtlety of this classificatory system lies in the fact that it is dynamic and not reduced to static duality. In yin there is always some yang, and in yang always some yin. . . . Yin and yang can be diagrammed as the poles of a continuous cyclic alternation. In this model, as in nature, the transitions between the alternative polarities take place gradually and in unbroken progression. All phenomena, including the parts of the body, are as-

signed yin and yang qualities, and hence man's place as a small
part of a great cosmic order is firmly established. (1980, 30)

The medicine of the yinyang system of correspondences is a
complex one, as shown in the following dialogue between the
legendary Yellow Emperor and his minister Chi Bo in *Huangdi
neijing:*

The Yellow Emperor asked . . . : I have heard it said that the
existence of man encompasses firmness and softness, weakness
and strength, short and long duration, as well as yin and yang
[regions]. I should like to discover in what relationship all this
stands to the methods of therapy.
[Chi Bo]: In yin there is yang, in yang there is yin. When one
is knowledgeable about yin and yang, he can apply needle treatments methodically. When the origins of illness have been
comprehended, the application of needles can be carried out on
the basis of the [proper] principles. Carefully assess the causes
of the affliction and the correspondences to the four seasons.
[The human body] consists of an inner region, comprising the
five depots [yin orbs] and the six palaces [yang orbs], and an
outer region, containing tendons, bones and skin. Thus yin and
yang [elements] are present in both inner and outer regions. In
the inner region the five palaces belong to the yin and the six
depots to the yang [sphere]. In the outer regions, the tendons
and bones belong to yin and the skin to yang. . . . If the illness
is located in the yang [sphere] it is called wind; if it is located in
the yin [sphere] it is called rheumatism. . . . If yin and yang
[regions] have been equally affected by illness, it is referred to
as wind rheumatism. . . . Illnesses that are manifest but do not
cause pain, belong to the yang category. If illnesses are not
manifest but cause pain, they belong to the yin category. If they
are not manifest but cause pain, the yang [sphere] is healthy
while the yin [region] has been damaged. In such cases, the yin
[sphere] should be treated as quickly as possible, while the yang
[sphere] is left alone. If [illnesses] are manifest but cause no
pain, the yin [sphere] is healthy but the yang [sphere] has been
damaged. [In such cases] treat the yang [sphere] as quickly as
possible and leave the yin [sphere] alone. When the yin and
yang [spheres] are agitated, when [an illness] is alternately
manifest and not manifest, and when, in addition, heart dis-
comfort occurs, it is said that the yin [sphere] is more severely

[afflicted] than the yang [sphere]. This signifies that neither the inner nor outer region alone has been affected by [a single illness]. [Such illnesses] do not remain manifest for long. (Unschuld 1985, 269–70)

Another key system of correspondences, and one that became fused with that of yin and yang, is *wuxing*, the "five evolutive phases." Table 2, below, illustrates the correspondence between the five phases, yinyang, and the organs of the body.

The five evolutive phases coexist in a cyclical, sequential relationship. Of the thirty-six different sequences, three are of particular importance in medicine. In the mutual production and mutual conquest sequences, the phases exist in harmony and account for normality and good health. (Porkert calls these sequences "physiological," in the sense that they are at work in all the normal functions of the living organism. In fact, they are instrumental in maintaining smooth and harmonious physiological operation.) In the violation sequence, the phases exist in disharmony and account for abnormality and ill health (Porkert 1974, 51–54). These three are best illustrated graphically (see Figures 1–3 below).

The two systems of correspondences discussed above—yinyang and five evolutive phases—constituted the basic theoretical core of classical Chinese medicine, around which many other theories were developed. In the most elemental sense, it can be said that when the forces of yinyang and five evolutive phases operate in harmony and perfect balance, a person en-

Table 2. Table of Correspondences

	Wood	Fire	Earth	Metal	Water
Yin orbs:	Liver	Heart	Spleen	Lungs	Kidneys
Yang orbs:	Gall Bladder	Small Intestines	Stomach	Large Intestines	Bladder
Sense:	Sight	Speech	Taste	Smell	Hearing
Orifice:	Eyes	Ears	Mouth	Nose	Anus
Taste:	Acid	Bitter	Sweet	Piquant	Salty
Emotions:	Anger	Joy	Worry	Grief	Fear

Adapted from Lock (1980), 32.

Figure 1
Mutual Production Sequence

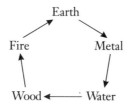

In this cycle, each evolutive phase produces the subsequent one. In his treatise "Luxuriant gems of the spring and autumn annals," the Han philosopher Dong Zhongshu wrote: "Wood is the beginning of the cycle of the Five [Evolutive Phases], Water is its end and Earth is its center. Such is the natural sequence. Wood produces Fire, Fire produces Earth, Earth produces Metal, Metal produces Water, and Water produces Wood." (Chan 1973, 279)

Figure 2
Mutual Conquest Sequence

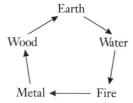

This sequence of mutual conquest was established by Zou Yan (305–240? B.C.) of the Yinyang School (Jia 1979, 31). He wrote: "Heaven gave him (Great Yu) with its Nine Categories. And the various virtues and their relations are regulated. . . . The first category is the Five [Evolutive Phases]; namely, Water, Fire, Wood, Metal, and Earth" (Chan 1973, 249). He thus established the domination of Fire by Water, Metal by Fire and so on.

Figure 3
Violation Sequence

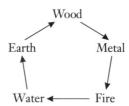

We see that the cycle depicted here is a reversal of that in Figure 2. Wood, instead of being checked by Metal, violates it; Metal, instead of being checked by Fire, violates it, and so on. Porkert characterizes the violation sequence as "pathological," in the sense that illness ensues when this sequence is in operation in the human body.

joys good health. Various forms of energy circulate through the body according to prescribed routes and function physiologically, keeping the person alive and well. Conversely, when these forces operate in disharmony and imbalance—that is, pathologically—one becomes ill.

Medical Explanations and Treatments for Madness

By the eighteenth century, the Chinese had already amassed a wealth of knowledge regarding madness. The volumes on medicine in the Qing encyclopedia *Qinding gujin tushu jicheng* (Synthesis of books and illustrations past and present), published in 1726, are a good index of this knowledge. The compilers of the encyclopedia collected most of the discourses on madness in the section called *diankuang*, but related materials can also be found in *qingzhi* (emotions) section. In this chapter, I will trace the evolution of Chinese medical explanations of madness chronologically, following closely the order established in the *Tushu jicheng*. The first entries in the collection consist of excerpts from the *Huangdi neijing*. Two major types of madness are identified: *dian* and *kuang*. Both conditions are explained in terms of yinyang imbalance. The *dian* condition is attributed to an overabundance of yin in a person's system, while the cause of *kuang* is assigned to an excess of yang. A passage in the *Neijing* contains a description of the behavior of a person who is afflicted with the *kuang* form of madness. The patient is easily startled by sudden, clapping sounds, is averse to heat, and exhibits a misanthropic tendency. During the crisis, when yang is most redundant, there is an uncontrollable desire to climb up high places, to chant, to sing, to disrobe in public, and to curse people (*YBCL* 1962, 1603–1604; Porkert 1974, 227).

In another passage of the *Huangdi neijing*, the legendary Yellow Emperor asks his minister Chi Bo what makes it possible for a *kuang* person to ascend heights that normally cannot be scaled. Chi Bo replies that because the four limbs are yang "bases," they become "firm" when yang is redundant. When the limbs are firm, a person can climb up high places without difficulty. The Yellow Emperor further asks why a *kuang* person tends to discard his or her clothing. Chi Bo explains that when yang is overabundant, the body becomes hot, thus stripping off garments is simply an attempt to cool off. The Yellow Emperor then asks why a *kuang* person curses people indiscriminately. Chi Bo explains that yang redundancy causes loss of the sense of propriety, thus leading a person to curse others, including close relatives. The commentary on this particular passage further explains that an overabundance of yang confuses the rational senses, thus causing a person to scold or curse others without regard for their status (*YBCL* 1962, 1600–1601).

A clear distinction between *dian* and *kuang* can be found in the Han medical classic *Nanjing* (Classic of difficult issues). According to one passage, at the onset of *kuang*, the patient hardly ever sleeps and is never hungry. The patient develops a superiority complex, thinking that he or she is noble and wise. The patient also loves to laugh and sing and create merriment, and is in perpetual motion. In stark contrast, at the onset of *dian*, the patient is very depressed and stares blankly ahead in a catatonic state. The author(s) of the *Nanjing* also believed that *dian* and *kuang* were caused by an imbalance in yinyang energies (ibid., 1604).

The Later Han period saw a major advance in medicine. Through the efforts of such great physicians as Zhang Ji (A.D. 145–220), medicine became more systematized and diagnoses based on clinical observations became firmly established as standard medical procedure. Zhang's major contribution to the understanding of disease etiology was his discourse on cold-related illnesses, *Shanghan lun* (On cold-induced bodily injuries). In this work, he firmly establishes cold as a major cause of many illnesses, including a form of madness peculiar to menstruating women. According to Zhang, a woman who succumbs to a cold-induced fever during her menstrual period is susceptible to an invasion of her uterus by "heat." As a result, the woman vacillates between lucidity and incoherence. During the day, she behaves in a normal fashion; by nightfall, however, she becomes "drowsy" and babbles incessantly as if possessed by a ghost. Fortunately, this is usually a temporary condition. Once the invading heat is discharged along with the menstrual blood, the woman will be restored to normalcy (Tseng 1973, 571).

Another great physician of the Later Han period was Hua Tuo (died ca. A.D. 208). He was a maverick physician, employing methods that were considered unorthodox by the standards of his day. Although he was an expert in herbal medicines, he was rather conservative in their use, limiting his prescriptions to a few well-tried formulas. His attitude toward the use of acupuncture was similar, employing the method on only a few acu-points in the body. For illnesses that neither his prescriptions nor acupuncture could cure, surgery was his preferred method of treatment (Jia 1979, 90–91). The medical text most commonly identified with Hua Tuo is the *Zhongzang jing* (Treasury classic). The Qing encyclopedia *Tushu jicheng*, for example, ascribes the work to him. In the section on *diankuang* (no distinction was made between *dian* and *kuang*), we find Hua Tuo advocating a noninterventionist approach to the treatment of madness:

> This illness originates in the six yang orbs and therefore belongs to the yang system. When yang energy erupts, it may course up or down, inward or downward, or it may become inverted. At the peak of its eruption, [a variety of symptoms are manifested]. There are patients who sing and laugh, or conversely, there are patients who weep sorrowfully. There are those who run about; those who moan and groan; those who belittle themselves; those who cannot sleep; those who cannot or will not talk. These varieties of symptoms all originate in the six yang orbs.
>
> [Understand the nature of the illness and facilitate that nature]. Do not contradict the patient's likes or dislikes, nor should you try to suppress their likes and dislikes (*YBCL* 1962, 1605).

The next major entry in this section is a piece written by the famous Tang physician Sun Simiao (581?–682). Like Hua Tuo before him, Sun was a maverick, shunning numerous invitations from the state to participate in government. His disdain for official appointments was probably due to his Daoist and

Buddhist inclinations (Jia 1979, 125). Sun was also an avid alchemist, tinkering frequently with the manufacture of the elixir of life. In one of his later works, the *Qianjin yifang* (Supplement to *A thousand golden remedies*), he even professed a belief in the efficacy of Daoist charms and incantations (Jia 1979, 129). Sun's interest in demonology was not unusual for the Tang period, yet he remained a practitioner of more orthodox methods. It was he who systematized the extremely useful "module system" in the art of acupuncture, making the task of determining the exact position of acu-points a much easier one. In Needham's opinion, if Sun "had done nothing else than this it would suffice to keep his memory undimmed among acupuncturists" (Needham and Lu 1980, 122). In his greatest work, the *Qianjin yaofang* (A thousand golden remedies), Sun describes many disease syndromes and offers precise treatments for each. For madness, Sun lists the following symptoms: refusal or unwillingness to talk or to make any sound; continuous chatter; uncontrolled singing and/or laughing; sitting or sleeping in street gutters or ditches; drinking and eating excreta and other filth; exhibitionism; roaming aimlessly day and night; and cursing people.

Sun Simiao's contribution was not so much his description of the symptoms of madness—many of the manifestations on his list had already been identified by earlier physicians—as his discussion of its pathology. In the *Qianjin yaofang*, Sun firmly establishes *feng* (wind) as a pathogenic agent for madness: "When *feng* enters the cardinal conduit of yang polarity (*yang jing*), *kuang* ensues; when *feng* enters the cardinal conduit of yin polarity (*yin jiang*), *dian* ensues" (*YBCL* 1962, 1606).

The revival of Confucianism in the Song epoch had significant impact on the evolution of medical thought in China. Medical theories based on naturalistic (as opposed to supernatural) concepts once again gained currency. The notion of *wuyun liuqi* (five phases of circulation and six climatic influences), for example, was introduced by Wang Bing during the Tang, but it was not until the Song that it gained the status of orthodoxy. P. Unschuld explains:

The five phases of circulation are five different time periods that together constitute a cycle. All are of equal duration, encompassing a total of one year. . . . Each of the five phases of circulation is associated with one of the Five Phases of Change. . . . The five phases of circulation ensure the orderly progression of seasons and formation of corresponding climatic conditions. . . . In addition to the five phases of circulation, the year was divided into a cycle of six climatic influences . . . which were also associated with yinyang duality and the Five Phases. . . .

The functions of the human organism, it was believed, are to a great extent determined by the influences that affect it during each season. [Liu Wenshu], who in 1099 published one of the best known works on the theory of the five phases of circulation and six climatic influences, went so far as to claim that each season was dominated by certain climatic influences that inevitably caused certain illnesses, giving rise to the concept of "illness caused by seasonal influence." (1985, 170–71)

One of the subscribers to the "cosmobiological" concepts of *wuyun liuqi* was the Jin period physician Liu Wansu (1110–1200). After years of study and observation, he concluded that among the six climatic influences—wind, dryness, dampness, cold, summer heat, and fire—the latter two had particular significance in the origin of illness. This notion informed his understanding of madness. In the *Hejian liushu* (The six books of Hejian), Liu discusses a manifestation of madness, *kuangyue:*

The word *kuang* means "raging, unpredictable wildness." The word *yue* means "perverting all rules of propriety and normal behavior."

Fire is wild and chaotic and murky. Water is clear and calm and smooth. Fire and Water are opposites. [In the human body], the kidneys correspond to the evolutive phase Water; they govern and check emotions and willpower (*zhi*). The heart corresponds to the evolutive phase Fire. It regulates the particular emotion joy. Since Fire and Water are opposites, when the evolutive phase Fire is resplendent, Water is depleted, and, so too, are the kidneys. When such a condition prevails, the patient loses control of his or her emotions and becomes *kuangyue.*

The commentary to the [*Huangdi*] *neijing* states: Excessive joy is a symptom of *dian;* excessive anger is a sympton of *kuang.* Indeed, joy is governed by the heart. When the heart is excessively hot, a person becomes *dian.* Anger is regulated by the liver. When Fire is strong, it overwhelms Metal to such a degree that Metal cannot check Wood [see Figure 2]. Consequently, the liver, which corresponds to the evolutive phase Wood, becomes strong. [When the liver is strong, a person becomes excessively angry and, therefore, *kuang*]. (*YBCL* 1962, 1608)

In the same work, he also explains why *kuang* patients have the propensity to curse and scold people indiscriminately:

Speech is the voice of the heart and, as such, abhors foul language. [The number for Water is six]; it is close to the Way and is therefore good. [The number of Fire is seven]; it is farther away from the Way than Water, and is therefore bad.

Water is clear and pure inside and not flashy outside; it abides by the shape of its vessel, it does not violate the taste, smell, or color of things. . . . Fire, [on the other hand], is bright and dazzling outside but murky inside; it burns and scorches all things. It makes things red, hot, bitter, charred.

Water is the child of Metal [see Figure 1]; it moistens and nourishes its mother. Fire is the child of Wood, but it harms its mother [see Figures 1, 3]. Thus there is the saying "Nothing nourishes things more than Water." Also, "Brilliant flame is like rebel troops." Therefore, we say when Water is above Fire, the situation is under control; when Water is beneath Fire, the situation is not under control. . . .

[Madness is a condition caused by redundancy of yang and exhaustion of yin]. Water is weak while Fire is strong. . . . When goodness is gone, evil becomes manifest. When [a person afflicted with this illness] scolds or curses people indiscriminately, or laughs and rages uncontrollably, it is all because of the heat generated by Fire. (*YBCL* 1962, 1608–9)

The predominant mode of treatment for madness was the use of herbal medicines or acupuncture or both. However, records show that a number of influential physicians also practiced "psychology" to treat their patients. Zhang Congzheng (1156–1228), for example, who was famous for his unorthodox

methods, was once called upon to treat a woman who had suddenly lost all her appetite for food. Moreover, she had frequent screaming fits and was dangerously violent. She was
given different medicines but none seemed to work. Feeling
desperate, her family overcame their initial reservations about
Zhang's methods and turned to him for help.

On the first day of the treatment, Zhang ordered two female
assistants to dress up in an outlandish fashion and sent them
on to his patient. When the sick woman saw the weirdly
garbed assistants, she burst into laughter for the first time in
many months. The next day, Zhang again sent his two assistants to see this patient, this time disguised as animals. Once
again, the sick woman laughed heartily. On the third day, he
arranged for the patient to witness his two collaborators wolf
down an exquisitely prepared meal. With her senses titillated
by the sight and smell of the feast, the sick woman recovered
her long-lost appetite for food. After several days of similar
treatment, she recovered from her long illness (*YBCL* 1962,
1649).

In another case, Zhang was asked to treat a man who had
become crazed after falling off a horse. The patient exhibited
almost all the classic symptoms of madness. He was incoherent, he could not distinguish between family and strangers, he
ran about stark naked, and he used foul language to scold and
curse people. Moreover, he became extraordinarily strong, so
that it required more than five men to subdue and tie him up.
His family did not immediately seek out Zhang Congzheng.
Instead, they repeatedly hired Daoist priests to perform rites
of exorcism on the patient, until they had almost exhausted all
their funds. It was at this point that they travelled two hundred
li to seek Zhang's help.

Zhang Congzheng devised an unusual contraption to treat
his patient. He buried a huge wheel in the ground, leaving
about twenty feet of its axle sticking out above the ground, and
a medium-sized wheel was placed on the open end of the axle.
Next, he tied his patient, lying prone and with his head facing
the ground, to the outer rim of the top wheel. After a gear device was attached, he hired a man to turn the entire assembly

"a thousand times." During the revolutions, the patient coughed up one or two *dou* of greenish fluid. This process was continued until the patient asked to be let down because he could tolerate it no longer. After he was untied and safely on the ground, he was given a large amount of ice water to drink. Another successful Zhang cure was rendered (*YBCL* 1962, 1649).

Zhang Congzheng was not always so unconventional in his methods. In another case, he was called upon to examine an old man, about sixty years of age, who had been mad for a number of years. His symptoms included a perpetual itch around his nose and mouth, which caused him to scratch himself almost incessantly. Upon interviewing the patient and his family, Zhang discovered that the old man had become ill years earlier, at about corvée labor tax time. Zhang figured the root cause of the illness to be vexation. As he explained it:

> The liver regulates the process of ideation, and the gall bladder governs the process of decision-making. [When the old man found that he did not have the funds to redeem his corvée tax, he became very agitated.] In such an agitated state, both the liver and gall bladder were activated. The liver produced many ideas but the gall bladder was indecisive. Thus, frustrations were pent up, and anger found no outlet. The energy of the E.P. [evolutive phase] Fire spread from the heart to the yang cardinal conduit . . . causing *kuang* madness.

Zhang placed his patient in a very warm room in order to induce him to sweat profusely. This treatment, used in conjunction with an herbal brew, was pronounced a success (*YBCL* 1962, 1649).

The great Yuan period physician Zhu Zhenheng (1281–1358) also believed that certain kinds of madness could not be treated successfully with herbal medicines alone. In his work *Danqi xinfa* (The methods of Danqi), Zhu identifies the seven emotions (joy, anger, desire, apprehension, fear, worry, and grief) as the principal causes of *dian* and *kuang*. Because emotion is the pathogenic agent, Zhu proposes using countering emotions to treat emotion-induced madness (*YBCL* 1962, 1610–11). His scheme is as follows:

Pathogenic agent	Neutralizing agents
anger	worry, apprehension
joy	anger, worry
desire	joy, anger
apprehension	desire, worry
fear	worry, apprehension
grief	apprehension, anger

Zhu Zhenheng's concept of using emotion to fight emotion gained many adherents during the Ming and Qing periods. The following is an interesting case that illustrates the use of Zhu's method: A young woman became extremely depressed after the death of her mother, with whom she had been especially close. She was lethargic and out of sorts, confining herself to bed almost all the time. Her worried husband hired a physician named Han Shiliang to look into her case. After examining the patient, Han told the husband that the woman's illness was caused by her yearning for her mother. Because it was an emotion-induced illness, it could not be treated with ordinary medicines. He recommended trying some "magic" instead.

After obtaining the husband's cooperation, Han bribed a medium and coached her thoroughly. He then asked the husband to suggest, innocently, to the young woman that since she missed her mother so much, it might not be a bad idea to hold a seance, so she could communicate with her mother. The young woman assented readily.

The medium delivered a sterling performance. Her impersonation of the dead woman was so perfect that the young patient was thoroughly taken in. When her "mother" appeared before her, she let loose her emotions and began to cry her heart out. However, her "mother" was in a vengeful mood.

"Stop crying at once!" the older woman ordered. "It was because of you that I died! Your fate blotted out mine! I have been wanting to avenge my death for some time. Your lingering illness is my doing. When I was alive, I was your mother. But now, I am your nemesis!" Upon hearing these heartless and vengeful words, the young woman turned her grief into anger. She hissed, "I became ill because I loved you and missed you so much. And yet you would do me harm. Why should I long for you any more!" With these words, her illness dissipated. Han noted, "This is an example of using emotion to treat illness" (*YBCL* 1962, 2101).

The placement of the case just described in the encyclopedia *Tushu jicheng* should be noted. The compilers chose to collect it under the category *qingzhi* (emotions) rather than *diankuang* (madness). This suggests that the interpretation of emotion-related illnesses was a problematic one for Qing experts. Some might consider them forms of madness, while others would not. It is possible that during the Qing period (and earlier), much as it is today, the diagnosis of madness depended on the physician's own experience and orientation. The following case illustrates this point:

One evening, while Wei Dexin and his wife were resting at a roadside inn, a band of robbers raided and set fire to the establishment. Needless to say, this unexpected attack frightened many patrons, including Wei's wife, who fell off her bed as a result. The woman had been extremely jumpy ever since, starting at even the slightest sound, so that the members of her household had to tiptoe around to avoid alarming her. A series of physicians were called upon to treat the woman. Almost to a man, they diagnosed her affliction as a form of emotion-induced madness (*xinbing*), and treated her accordingly. However, none of them was able to render a cure. The woman's condition thus persisted for many months, until Wei overcame his dislike for Zhang Congzheng and invited him to take up the case.

Zhang dismissed the diagnoses of the other physicians. In his opinion, the woman was suffering from the pathological consequences of fright, not madness. The frightful experience of the bandit raid had injured her gall bladder, which is a yang orb that regulates a person's courage. Characteristically, he opted for a non-medicinal method of treatment. He summoned two maid servants and instructed them to hold their mistress's hands firmly against the back of a chair. He placed a table in front of the patient and asked her to keep her eyes focused on it. He then picked up a piece of wood and hit the table with it, making a loud noise. The woman jumped up in fright at the sound.

Zhang said to the woman, "You saw me hit the table with the piece of wood, so why were you frightened?" After a short while, when the woman had regained her composure, he hit the table again, stopping when the woman once again became very frightened. He repeated this procedure about five more times, simultaneously ordering some servants to make scratching sounds on the window behind the woman's back, so as to surround her with different kinds of sound. Gradually, she became less easily startled. She even had the composure to ask Zhang to explain his method. Quoting from the *Huangdi neijing*, Zhang said, "It has been written, 'Treat a frightened person with means that placate or pacify (*ping*).' Since *ping* also means 'ordinary' (*pingchang*), it is only appropriate that I render ordinary [things that] disturb or frighten you. Once you have become used to them, you will no longer be easily alarmed by them."

That same evening, Zhang sent someone to knock on the woman's bedroom window all night long, in order to reinforce the conditioning that he had started earlier that day. This unusual approach proved to be very effective, and not even claps of thunder could scare the woman out of her wits any more. As a postscript, Zhang noted that the woman's husband became a lifelong admirer of his methods. He took it upon himself to strike anyone who dared to question or ridicule Zhang's expertise (*YBCL* 1962, 2160).

During the Ming period, a self-confident and self-centered attitude presided over the quest for knowledge. This attitude is summed up very well in the words of the Ming philosopher Chen Xianzhang (1428–1500): "Is there any idea not in one's own mind? Why is it necessary to copy the ancients?" (Jen 1970, 74). The conviction that the individual—more specifically, his mind alone—is the measure of all things encouraged skepticism and a healthy unwillingness to accept any theory at face value. In the world of medicine, this conviction brought about a period of unprecedented intellectual ferment:

> The climate fostered by such a philosophy persisted through the Ming to the conclusion of the [Qing] era, stimulating an extremely fruitful period in medical thought that lasted more than four centuries. But it was a fruitfulness that led to an even greater divergence of opinion; decade after decade saw new theories proposed and older views criticized, with no single approach being able to achieve sufficient authority to displace the others. It is a characteristic feature of this period that its insights remained tied to individual scholars, and that no single approach was sufficiently plausible to convince the majority of medical practitioners and achieve, even temporarily, the position of a generally recognized doctrine. (Unschuld 1985, 197)

During the Ming, there emerged a school, known commonly as the Warmth-restoring School (*wenbu pai*), which challenged the orthodoxy established by such medical greats as Zhang Ji, Liu Wansu, and Zhu Zhenheng. Both Zhang and Liu regarded "heat" as a pathogenic agent. Zhu Zhenheng, in his study of emotion-induced illnesses, had also established the theory that the human body houses a kind of energy called *xianghuo* (ministerial fire) which can become harmful when it is aroused by emotions or passions. Zhang, Liu, and Zhu all advocated the use of heat purgatives to combat illness. Adherents of the Warmth-restoring School, on the other hand, subscribed to a radically different theory of disease causation. While they did not deny that some illnesses could be caused by "heat," and therefore should be treated with heat purgatives, they were convinced that in most cases, heat deficiency was actually the principal pathogenic factor. They therefore recommended the use of warmth-restoring medicines to combat disease (Jia 1979, 214–15).

One of the most prominent figures in this school was Zhang Jiebin (1563–1640), the author of the famous treatise *Jingyue chuanshu* (The complete works of Jingyue). Zhang was initially a follower of the teachings of Zhu Zhenheng and Liu Wansu, but around the age of forty, after having accumulated years of observation and experience, he concluded that the old masters' theories concerning disease causation were untenable. Specifically, he rejected the notion that a pathological surplus of yang influences is frequently present in the body. He wrote:

> The only possibility one need fear in regard to the yang component is that it might be insufficiently developed and, in the case of the yin component, that it might be overly developed. The yin component is, however, by itself incapable of reaching a state of excess; for this it requires a deficiency of yang [influences]. The animation of all things is dependent upon yang [influences]; similarly the death of all living beings is dependent upon yang influences. But the yang [influences] themselves do not kill, for life itself arises where yang influences are present. Death occurs where yang [influences] fail to appear! (Unschuld 1985, 200)

Although Zhang rejected the idea that the human body could accumulate an excess of yang influences, he nonetheless elected not to challenge the ancient explanation that the *kuang* form of madness was caused by an excess of yang. However, in the *Jingyue chuanshu*, he warns of the danger of lumping *dian* and *kuang* together as a single, heat-induced disease. He cautions physicians not to use reflexively heat purgatives to treat madness. It is absolutely imperative, he insists, that they first determine whether the illness is of a yin or yang nature before prescribing medicine for the patient (*YBCL* 1962, 1618–21).

There remained, during the Ming-Qing period, an influential school of physicians who continued to acknowledge the validity of the principal ideas of such Song-Yuan masters as Zhu Zhenheng and Dai Sigong. They emphasized the importance of heat purgatives, both in maintaining good health and in combating illness. Many of the prominent physicians of the Qing period belonged to this school of thought, which, because of its uncompromising criticisms of the warmth-restorationists (especially Zhang Jiebin), was sometimes referred to as the Anti-Warmth-restoring School (Jia 1979, 215–16).

One of the "heat purgers" was the early Qing physician Chen Shiduo (ca. 1687). Chen was best known for his work on women's medical problems, but he had also written extensively on the subject of insanity. In his most noteworthy work, *Shishi bilu* (Confidential records of the stone room), Chen discusses two unusual forms of madness: *huadian* (literally, "flower madness") and *ai* (usually translated as "idiocy"). Chen characterizes *huadian* as the pathological outcome of unrequited love, manifested only in women. A woman who is afflicted with this condition loses her sense of propriety or shame. She thinks that all men are fair game and refuses to let go of those she encounters. Chen recommends giving the patient a concoction of herbs which douses the "fire" that rages inside her. Force it down her throat if necessary, he writes, even if this means incurring her wrath. She will soon become drowsy and fall asleep. Upon awakening, she will become so ashamed of herself that she will hide in her room for three days. She is on her way to recovery (*YBCL* 1962, 1622).

The illness that Chen identified as *ai* is not idiocy. The patient "acts like a befuddled fool" and behaves in a very bizarre manner:

> The patient sometimes sleeps for several days and several nights in a row without waking, but, equally likely, he may stay awake for several days and several nights in a row without sleeping. He sometimes sews tightly together the clothes he is wearing; he sometimes takes other people's things and hides them in a secret place. He cannot converse coherently, for his mind tends to wander. When he talks to himself, it is usually in a very low, sobbing voice. He usually refuses to eat any food that is offered him, yet, when he is denied food, he stuffs himself happily with charcoal.

Chen's recommendation for a cure was just as bizarre as the malady itself:

> First, coax the patient into drinking about half a bowl of an herbal brew (to dissipate the pent-up phlegm in the patient's chest). Offering the patient a piece of charcoal along with the medicine usually succeeds in making him cooperate. This process must be repeated again later in the day. The second dose of medicine should induce the patient to become drowsy and fall into a deep slumber that may last several days.

Next, remove and burn the patient's entire wardrobe, his blankets, and his mattress. It is to be expected that the patient, when he finally awakens, will protest such a drastic measure, but there is no need to heed his complaints.

It is necessary at this point to administer a third dose of medicine. Since the patient will be in a very foul mood, this will not be an easy task; the use of force may be called for. A strong person may have to be enlisted to force the medicine down the patient's throat. Exhausted by his furious, but ineffective, struggle against his rough treatment, the patient will fall into a deep sleep again. This slumber will last several hours, during which time fresh clothes and new bedding should be prepared. Family members should also be gathered in the patient's room to await his awakening.

When the patient awakens and finds himself surrounded by his relatives, he will weep as though he has finally recognized the cause of his problem; he will rant about ghosts and demons. His relatives should try to comfort him with soothing words, letting him know that someone has already chased the demons away and that there is no need for him to worry anymore. Having been thus reassured, the patient will recover from his affliction. (*YBCL* 1962, 1623)

A clear statement of Chen Shiduo's medical orientation is found in the section "Treatments for Madness" in the *Shishi bilu*:

The majority of *kuang* cases are "hot" diseases. The patient climbs up high places and sings; discards his or her clothing and runs about naked; jumps into bodies of water; scolds, curses, and threatens to kill people. . . . A *kuang* patient who only scolds people, who is never thirsty and who always refuses to drink water . . . is suffering from a fever that is caused by pent up *qi* (energy) as well as anger that has not been vented. . . .

A patient who is chronically *kuang*, who brandishes a sharp weapon and [threatens] to kill people, who insults officials, who does not recognize kinfolk, who does not know his or her children, who delights in water, [or] who becomes furious at the sight of food, is suffering from an illness that is caused by an exhaustion of the energy of the heart. The pathogenic agent, heat, takes advantage of this exhaustion to invade the body, thereby causing the illness. (*YBCL* 1962, 1524–25)

The attribution of *kuang* to excessive yang, coupled with the association of yang with male qualities, contributed to the notion that an excessively voracious sexual appetite was a symptom of the *kuang* form of madness. The famous Qing physician Wu Jutong (active during the late Qianlong and early Jiaqing periods) was once asked to treat a man who had been suffering from *kuang* madness for over seven years. When Wu saw his patient for the first time, he found him in a deplorable state. The poor man was stark naked, his wasted body completely covered with filth and grime. Although his hands and feet were chained and fettered, he still managed to smash everything within his reach. Besides being very violent, the patient also had an insatiable sexual appetite, demanding to have intercourse with a woman every day. He would broadcast this need with screams and loud wails. His family had no choice but to force his concubines to satisfy his needs. Wu concluded that the sick man had too much yang in his system. He prescribed an extremely bitter medicine to purge the heat from the patient's system. This treatment was effective and the patient recovered fully from his long illness (Qin 1959, 22–23).

A similar case was recorded by another famous Qing physician, Wang Mengying (mid-nineteenth century):

> Old Man Li, when he was in his seventies, expressed a desire to acquire a concubine. Because of his advanced age, his family dared not acquiesce to his desire. Old Man Li became so frustrated that he eventually became mad [*kuang*]. The family hired a succession of physicians to treat him, but because they all used warmth-restoratives, the old man's condition only worsened. Finally, they turned to me for help.
>
> The old man's pulse was extremely strong. His face was flushed, and he drooled uncontrollably. His physical strength was just like a young man's. I explained to his family that the old man's problem was caused by an overabundance of yang.
>
> The other physicians had completely failed to realize that a man over fifty years of age begins to lose his yin essence, and gradually accumulates an excess of yang. As with all things in nature, fire rages when yin is exhausted. I prescribed some

"cooling" medicines for the old man. I also ordered his family to give him huge quantities of pear juice, a natural coolant. In the end, all my efforts were for naught. Someone [contrary to my advice] gave the old man some ginger broth (a very yang drink). Consequently, he suffered a relapse. This time, not even I could cure him. (Wang 1957, 46)

Heat purgers firmly believed that the indiscriminate use of warmth-restoring medicines was extremely dangerous; so, too, was excessive consumption of yang or "hot" foods, especially when a person's physiological processes already showed signs of yang redundancy. The following case, taken from the treatise *Weisheng baojian*, illustrates this point of view:

A male servant suddenly became mad (*kuang*) one day. He had all the familiar symptoms. For instance, he tore off all his clothes and ran wildly about stark naked, he screamed and yelled at people without any provocation, and he could not distinguish between strangers and kin. He also had a great thirst for milk (a "hot" drink), which he tried to share with whoever crossed his path. Many people believed that he had been bewitched, so a shaman was hired to exorcize the demons. However, not only did the young man fail to benefit from the shaman's ministrations, but his condition actually grew steadily worse. This was in large part because he continued to drink huge quantities of milk, which caused him to become constipated. Moreover, he had also been eating mutton, a very "hot" food. In other words, his diet compounded his illness. Finally, a physician correctly diagnosed his problem and prescribed a laxative to purge his system of the excess heat that had been stored up for so long. The following morning, the physician found that the patient's pulse and body temperature were normal, and that all symptoms of his illness had disappeared (*YBCL* 1962, 1650).

The coexistence of two radically different schools did not lead to paralyzing confusion for practitioners of Chinese medicine. Unschuld explains this very well:

Although we may witness, in the literature, sufficient traces of heated argumentations between the schools propagating opposing views, after a while the issue was resolved neither in a dialectical sense in that a more advanced synthesis was created out of thesis and antithesis nor in a (Kuhnian) revolutionary sense in that a more recent paradigm achieved prevalence and dominated a subsequent era of "normal science" until it was replaced by the next revolutionary paradigm. The unique feature of the Chinese situation—and this should receive more attention from historians and philosophers of science—is the continuous tendency toward a syncretism of all ideas that exist (within accepted limits). Somehow a way was always found in China to reconcile opposing views and to build bridges—fragile as they may appear to the outside observer—permitting thinkers and practitioners to employ liberally all the concepts available, as long as they were not regarded as destructive to society. (1985, 57–58)

Factional affiliations notwithstanding, Chinese physicians shared a common language. Diseases were explained in terms of disharmony and imbalance; the goal of medicine was to restore and maintain harmony and balance. Illnesses caused by yang redundancy, for example, were treated with medicines or procedures that would rid the system of the excess yang energy and restore the depleted yin to healthy levels. Similarly, "hot" diseases were combated with "cooling" medicines, and "cold" diseases were treated with "warming" medicines.

Regardless of their orientation, Chinese physicians universally understood the many forms of madness to be organic disorders, and the language used to explain the pathology of *dian* and *kuang* was not at all different from that used to explain other illnesses. The notion that madness could be a *mental* illness was never advanced, not even by those who saw a distinct relationship between emotions and madness. The holistic approach of classical Chinese medicine has made the distinction between "physical" and "mental" alien to the Chinese experience. However, as we have seen in the preceding discussion, behavioral disorders were certainly recognized—for example, the classic symptoms of *kuang* madness—but only as manifestations of physiological dysfunctions.

Precisely because madness was regarded as an organic disorder, it carried no stigma as far as the medical community was concerned. There is no reference in the medical literature to moral turpitude as a cause of madness. This is in marked contrast to late eighteenth- and early nineteenth-century England, where a connection between madness and morality was made. Such a connection encouraged the evolution of a specialized approach to treatment that occupied the middle ground between medicine and such religious notions as possession by the devil. The York Retreat, founded by the Quakers in 1792, was a notable showcase for the moral management approach (see Digby 1985). Later in the nineteenth century, with the growing professionalization of medicine, physicians moved to appropriate moral management for themselves, and eventually succeeded in monopolizing the treatment of madness. In China, such social and professional dynamics did not come into play.

Physicians did not monopolize the management of illness in China. As the incident presented at the beginning of this chapter shows, sick people also used home remedies, prayers, sacrifices, restitutions, and even rites of exorcism. The recourse chosen at a particular time depended on the explanation adopted by the sick and their families. As Ilza Veith indicates, popular beliefs regarding madness centered around supernatural causes (1963, 139). Three phenomena in particular were most commonly accepted as causes of madness: retribution for sinful deeds, possession by malevolent spirits, and separation of the soul from the body. The way a mad person was received in the community depended in large part on the attributed cause of the illness. Madness resulting from sin or from spirit possession did not invite feelings of magnanimity from others. Thus madness in the popular perception carried with it a certain stigma.

Retribution for Sins

According to Wolfram Eberhard, the notion of sin—that is, a violation of a divine code—is not indigenous to China. This concept did not appear in the popular mind until the introduction of Buddhism to China and its subsequent popularization into a folk religion. Folk Buddhism introduced not only the notion of sin but also its companion, divine retribution (see Eberhard 1967, chap. 1). The practical Chinese developed a rather simple device to help them allay the wrath of the gods. Printed "writs of pardon" could be purchased by fearful sinners at shops which specialized in religious paraphernalia. However, for these writs to be efficacious, the services of Buddhist or Daoist priests were usually required. Henri Doré described a typical response:

> The sinner, who wishes to obtain the pardon of his sins, begs the Buddhist or [Daoist] priests to pray for him, or even fast in his behalf, if he pays them for so doing. The Buddhist priests then write his name on the writ of pardon, taking care to indicate the year, month and day, in which the favour is granted. The document is then burnt, and thus forwarded to the ruler of Hades. The sins of the supplicant, in whose behalf the document was granted, and of which a list was inscribed on the writ, are henceforth deemed effaced. (Doré 1966, 5:524–25)

A rich body of literature exists that details horrifying consequences of sinful conduct. I have selected several tales from the Qing collection *Guobao wenjian lu* (Anthology of tales of retribution) and Pu Songling's *Liaozhai zhiyi* (Stories from a strange studio) to illustrate the variety of misdeeds that could bring about disastrous consequences, including madness:

> On the grounds of Tianning Temple in Ningbo was a deserted shrine where a statue of the deity Guandi was housed. One day, two young men, taking advantage of the secluded location, committed a homosexual act right in front of the statue. This immediately brought forth a ferocious response from Guandi. "How dare you defile this temple!" he roared. "You shall die for this!"
> The frightened youths were able to pull up their pants, but the shock was so great that they began to scream uncontrollably, attracting a huge crowd to the usually deserted shrine. After a short while, the parents of the two youths caught wind of the incident and hurried to the shrine to offer a pledge to

Guandi that they would arrange for a play to be performed as an atonement for their sons' sin. Guandi's anger subsided, and the screaming fit finally came to an end. However, the two youths remained in a daze for another month. (*Guobao wenjian lu*, in *BXD* 1974, 3d ser., 6606)

The sin that occasioned the fit of temporary madness—uncontrolled screaming was one of the classic symptoms of madness—was the homosexual act, aggravated by the fact that it was performed before the statue of Guandi. As was noted in Chapter One, homophobia in China was a Qing development. Male homosexuality did not become a felony until later when the Qing government introduced the male rape law and at the same time criminalized sodomy between consenting adults.

Another sin that from the point of view of devout Buddhists warranted divine retribution was the taking of life, as the following story shows:

Once upon a time, there lived a butcher. He was very adept with the knife and for good reasons too, for his family had been in the business for generations. Although he and his wife led a comfortable life—business was very good—they were not completely happy, for even after many years of marriage, they had not yet been blessed with a son and heir.

There was something else too that bothered the butcher. He had inexplicably begun to put on weight, so much so that his neck became a mass of fat and his eyes were but two sunken holes in his grotesquely fleshy face. In other words, he was beginning to look more and more like a pig!

One day, he came down with a strange illness that caused him to grunt like a pig at frequent intervals. On the seventh day of his illness, he suddenly lost his mind. He climbed over a bridge, grunted three times, and then threw himself into the river. His body was never recovered. Shortly after his suicide, his wife suffered a miscarriage. Eventually, she remarried, forsaking his lineage forever. (*Guobao wenjian lu*, in BXD 1974, 3d ser., 6607)

The butcher's sin was his occupation, and his punishment was severe indeed. Every conceivable calamity that could befall a Chinese befell him. He became insane and took his own life. His widow suffered a miscarriage shortly after his death and subsequently remarried, thus ensuring that there would not be anyone to carry on his family name and perpetuate ancestral sacrifices. He and his ancestors were destined to be hungry ghosts who must roam endlessly in search of food. So even his forbears were posthumously punished.

In family- and lineage-conscious China, perpetuation of the descent line was of paramount concern. Thus, to cause the termination of someone's family line was considered an abominable sin. The following story from Pu Songling's *Liaozhai zhiyi* depicts a greedy man who was afflicted with madness for committing such a sin:

> A certain man, coveting the property of his heirless uncle, agreed to become the uncle's adopted son. After the older man's death, however, he reneged on his agreement, thus in effect ending his uncle's descent line.
>
> This man had another uncle who also had no sons; once again he agreed to adoption and once again, he renounced the agreement after his uncle's death. He had thus consolidated his two uncles' estates into his own.
>
> One day, quite suddenly, this man became raving mad. He kept muttering to himself, "So you want to be rich and still live, eh?" All the while, he carved slivers of flesh from his own body and cast them onto the ground. Unable to control himself, he then plunged the knife into his abdomen and disemboweled himself. Soon after his death, his son also died and his estate fell into the hands of others. (Pu 1976, 755)

In many tales of retribution, the sudden onset of madness was, although not the ultimate punishment, part of a chain of events that culminated in the sinner's death, usually by his or her own hand. Thus, social stigma could result when a person suddenly became deranged, and the condition was interpreted by others as retribution for some sinful deed.

Possession

Belief in demons and spirits has a very ancient history in China. The spirits were believed to dwell in myriad abodes.

They could be found in water, trees, animals, rocks, soil, graves, eaves of houses, and even sculptures. These demons and spirits, when not properly appeased or placated, could cause a host of misfortunes for human beings—for example, madness, chronic illness, suicide, and other seemingly inexplicable phenomena. Perhaps the most dreaded of all demonic spirits were the spirits of the dead, especially those belonging to individuals who had died violent deaths and those who had been denied proper burial. The following tale, recorded in the Qing collection *Tan yi* (Discourses on unusual happenings), describes the vicissitudes of a young woman who was possessed by the ghost of a murdered woman:

> One year in July, my sister suddenly came down with a high fever. As the fever lingered on she began to act rather strangely, as if she had suffered a terrible wrong. But although she was obviously hurting inside she refused to tell anyone the reasons for her unhappiness. Some of my servants, being natives of Guangdong and therefore very superstitious, suggested that her illness was caused by a ghost and urged me to consult a shaman. I rejected their recommendation because I was certain that my sister's illness was of an organic nature.
>
> However, her condition continued to worsen. One night, she even tried to hang herself. Luckily, she was discovered in the nick of time. Six days later, she tried to kill herself again by jabbing an acupuncture needle into her own heart. At first, we did not know how to save her but we finally settled on moxibustion. As we were applying moxa to the wound, my sister's voice suddenly changed to that of another woman. We immediately asked who it was that was speaking through my sister. The voice answered, "My name is Ho. I was killed by Guangdong bandits who later threw my body into a river. My spirit has since been roaming from place to place." (*Tan yi*, in *BXD* 1974, 4th ser., 5641)

Ancestors, too, could become malevolent spirits to haunt their descendants. Yuan Mei's collection of anecdotes and supernatural tales, *Zi bu yu* (Matters Confucius refused to talk about), contains the following short account: The grandmother of a gravely ill young man appeared in his dream to tell him that if he wanted to get well he should take ginseng. When he related the dream to his doctor, the latter warned him emphatically that ginseng was absolutely harmful for him and that he should not try it. However, the grandmother once again appeared in the young man's dream, urging him once more to take ginseng. She even told him where he could locate the medicinal plant. He followed her instructions and, against his doctors advice, ate the ginseng. As a result, in the middle of the night, he became raving mad and died (*Zi bu yu*, in *BXD* 1974, 2d ser., 5574).

In a number of spirit-possession tales, there seems to be a definite link between sexual awakening and madness. The following story, involving a young scholar and a turtle spirit, is one example:

When Shu Xindao was a young man he came under the thrall of a turtle spirit. It started one evening when Shu was studying alone in his room. A woman suddenly appeared before him and confessed to him that she had been a secret admirer and would like to share her life with him. She was a good match for Shu, being quite skilled in the literary arts as well as in sewing. They thus spent about a month or so together, unbeknownst to the rest of Shu's family.

One day, Shu's personal servant happened to overhear him talking with someone. He said to himself, "Master must be cavorting with a prostitute. If this should ever come to light, I would be in serious trouble!" But he confided his suspicions to another servant, who in turn leaked the information to others. This was how Shu's family found out about the incident.

One evening, Shu's brothers and sisters dropped in on him unannounced. The startled woman scurried about the room and then disappeared from sight. Shu was heartbroken. "I will never be able to see her again!" he wailed. Seeing him thus the others left him alone and closed the door behind them. The woman reappeared. She was a sorry sight! She was dripping wet, her hair was completely disheveled and her feet were bare. Between taking huge gulps of air, the woman blurted out that she had fallen into the sea. Fortunately, because the water was not too deep, she had not drowned. Shu Xindao was deeply moved. He boiled some water for her, gave her a bath, and then the couple went to bed together. They thus resumed their illicit relationship.

The deeper Shu became involved with the woman, the more his health suffered. He became absentminded and disoriented, and he lost all interest in food. [These were all classic symptoms of madness, and well-documented in medical texts.] Convinced that he had become possessed by an evil spirit, his family sought the aid of Zhu Yancheng, a Daoist exorcist. Once he was presented the particulars of the case, Zhu was certain that the malevolent agent was the spirit of a turtle. He said, "The evil influences have entered the liver as well as the spleen. Such a condition cannot be cured by religious charms alone." He then set off to the Shu residence to combat the evil spirit in his own way.

The turtle spirit/woman sensed the imminent threat to her well-being. She started sobbing and looked absolutely pitiful, moving Shu to implore her to explain the reason for her distress. Still sobbing, she said, "A Daoist priest is coming tomorrow to wreck everything for me. I have to leave." Shu Xindao begged her to stay. But it was to no avail, for she took her leave that same day.

The Daoist arrived the following day and immediately went about his business. He asked the Shu family to borrow a huge wok from a nearby monastery and to heat up twenty catties of oil in it. He went to the edge of the pond and told everyone present that he would exorcize the turtle spirit right before their eyes. He burned several pieces of charms and summoned his supernatural army to chase the evil spirit from its hiding place at the bottom of the pond. Shortly afterward, the water in the pond became agitated and a strange creature surfaced from the bottom. It was a giant white turtle! And it nodded its head as if it were begging for its life. But instead it crawled toward the gigantic wok of hot oil and immersed itself in it. The bystanders all shuddered with horror at the terrible sight. Shu Xindao was grief-stricken. "You have cooked my beloved!" he sobbed.

The Daoist turned to Shu's family and said to them, "When the oil has cooled down sufficiently, take the turtle out, crack open its shell, and separate the meat from the bones. Lay everything out in the sun to dry thoroughly. I repeat, thoroughly! Grind the pieces up with ginseng, fir fungus, and dragon bones.

The mixture is a very good restorative and should be given to the patient twice a day, in the morning and at night, until you have used it all up. Be sure, however, not to let him know what you are giving him or he will surely refuse the medicine." The family did as they were told and just as the Daoist had predicted, Shu Xindao recovered fully from his affliction. (*Wuyao zhi*, in *BXD* 1974, 5th ser., 4578–80)

Young women, particularly those on the verge of marriage, seemed to be especially susceptible to the lecherous attention of malevolent spirits, and they often became temporarily insane as a result. The following are two examples:

A young bride, on her wedding day, was getting ready to board the bridal palanquin when she suddenly became raving mad. She rushed out of her father's house and started to beat up people who had gathered around the house for the occasion. She kept saying these words to herself: "I won't marry an ordinary person. I just won't!" A shaman was summoned. He led the young woman to the bank of the river, took out his drum, and began beating on it while reciting a chant at the same time. Some skeptics among the crowd thought that it was all hocuspocus.

The next day, however, a green snake slithered out from nowhere. The shaman immediately drove a huge nail through its head. Several hours later, around noon, a huge tortoise crawled out of the river and surrendered itself to the shaman. The exorcist scribbled a few words on the tortoise's head and sent it back to the river. At dusk, a giant white water lizard surfaced from the bottom of the river, with the tortoise in hot pursuit. Risking certain death, the lizard made its way to the young woman's room to bid her farewell. The woman was heartbroken. But gradually, she regained her senses and grew shameful about the entire incident.

The shaman later explained to the curious witnesses that the green snake was a messenger, the tortoise was the matchmaker, and the lizard was to be the young woman's bridegroom. All three creatures were subsequently killed. (*Wuyao zhi*, in *BXD* 1974, 5th ser., 4580–81)

Scholar Chen was blessed with a beautiful daughter. When she reached the marriageable age, Chen began preparations to arrange a match for her. It was at this time, however, that the young woman fell under the spell of an evil spirit and subsequently lost her rational senses. Since Chen was quite well off, he spared no expense trying one shaman after another to effect a cure for his dear daughter. It was all in vain. One year went by and the young woman's condition remained unchanged.

It so happened that one night, their neighbor had his curiosity aroused by the sound of the woman's laughter. He decided to peer over the wall for a good look. In order to do so, he had to climb on the stone statue of a lion which graced Chen's front gate. As he straightened up on the back of the statue, the woman suddenly turned toward him and growled, "I have never interfered with your affairs, why do you plague me so?"

It dawned on the neighbor that the spirit which inhabited the stone lion was the cause of the woman's year-long affliction. He informed Chen of his discovery and further recommended that the stone lion be smashed and the pieces dumped into the river. Chen carried out his recommendations and shortly afterward his daughter recovered from her illness. (*Wuyao zhi*, in *BXD* 1974, 5th ser., 4605)

The stories presented above are rich not only with clues concerning popular conceptions of madness but attitudes toward sexuality as well. They suggest, first of all, a high level of sexual anxiety. The two young women, of marriageable age, suddenly became insane around the time of betrothal. Were they so fearful of marital sexual relations that they became crazed? The fact that their strange afflictions are explained in terms of sexual possession by lecherous spirits is significant, for it hints at the latent sexual nature of their problems. Ilza Veith, too, has noticed the phenomenon of young women becoming insane upon reaching or passing marriageable age. However, she has a different interpretation, attributing the condition to malevolent intervention of ancestral spirits: "Especially vulnerable to ancestral mischief were young girls whose marriageable age had passed without the appearance of a suitable husband. Forever deprived of a proper place in society, they tended to believe themselves haunted and to become emotionally unbalanced. In some the delusion eventually led to insanity" (1963, 144).

Spirit possession as an explanation for madness did not seem to stigmatize insanity in the same way as did the concept of divine retribution. The afflicted persons were often seen as hapless victims of malevolent and capricious spirits and, as such, they were to be pitied rather than ostracized. At the same time, however, it was perhaps inevitable that some might question why certain individuals were more susceptible to possession than others. Could it be that there was something about them that made them ideal hosts for malevolent spirits? In the popular imagination, then, a connection between moral turpitude and madness could be established.

Whatever the assigned cause of the condition might be, one thing is certain: it was left to the family to provide the necessary care for the afflicted individual. As was noted earlier in this chapter, unlike England or France, especially in the nineteenth century, there were no special institutions or asylums in China set up for the care and confinement of lunatics. A few homeless or otherwise destitute insane people might have found accommodations in hospitals set up by Buddhist temples, but for those with families, care was typically provided by their kin.

A number of foreigners who lived in China during the late nineteenth and early twentieth centuries noted with dismay the "pitiable" condition of the insane in China. For example, Dr. J. L. McCartney lamented that mental patients constituted "a very helpless class" in China. He wrote with undisguised horror that if the insane were caught doing anything wrong, they were arrested and thrown in prison and treated as if they were criminals. Those who stayed out of trouble were frequently mocked and laughed at and even stoned by those they did not know. Their families, too, treated them very shabbily, sometimes regarding them as strangers and confining them in dark rooms by themselves (Lamson 1935, 416–17). John H. Gray offered another eyewitness account:

> In China there are no lunatic asylums. Violent lunatics are kept manacled in dark, inner rooms in their own houses. Where the family is poor, the want of asylums entails great hardship. I have seen a lunatic lying by the side of the highway bound hand and foot, without a creature near him to render him the slightest as-

sistance. When at large he had manifested violence, and his un-feeling countrymen, instead of conveying him where he might be securely kept, bound him hand and foot, and left him lying by the wayside. On another occasion, I saw a female lunatic traversing the streets of Canton in a state of nudity. The poor woman was being pursued by a number of lads, who were beat-ing her unmercifully with rods. On being expostulated by some Europeans, they coolly replied that she was possessed by a devil, and well-deserved her treatment. The unfortunate crea-ture took shelter in the ruins of a Danish factory, which had been destroyed at the commencement of the war in 1856. After remaining there for some days she was removed, at the expense of three or four European merchants, to a place of comfort and security. Lunatics who are not violent, are allowed to go at large. (Gray 1878, 2:55)

Not all Chinese were unsympathetic to the plight of the in-sane. I have come across a number of didactic tales whose pur-pose was to educate readers not to poke fun at people who ap-peared to be insane. In many of these stories, the mad person who had been ridiculed turned out to be an immortal. The fol-lowing story appeared in the anthology *Shenxian biji jinghua* (The best of stories about immortals):

One day during the Jiaqing period, a plain-looking peasant woman and her infant son walked into a busy shop to purchase some goods. When it came time to pay the shop clerk, the woman placed her son on the counter so she could count out the money to pay her bill. Now, this little boy was absolutely filthy. He was sweaty and covered with grime and dirt. His body odor was such that one could lose one's appetite for three days! Anyway, while his mother was busy counting her money, this little kid suddenly let loose his bowels and made a mess of the counter. The offending odor was utterly unbearable! The flustered clerk scolded the woman and ordered her to clean up the mess. The woman smiled good-naturedly and apologized, "It's all my son's fault. Don't worry, I'll just ask him to eat it all up."
    True to her words, the woman scooped up the mess with her fingers and fed it to her son, mouthful by the mouthful. The stupid child did not mind it at all. In fact, he seemed to enjoy

himself thoroughly. Everyone in the shop snickered at the crazy woman and her idiotic son. Before too long, all that was left of the mess was a few smudges here and there. But the woman, instead of telling the clerk that she was through with her cleaning task, stared at the smudges for a little while and proceeded to lick the counter clean! When that was done the woman picked up her son and walked out of the shop.

When they were out of sight, someone in the shop noticed a strange fragrance that seemed to emanate from the spot on the counter where the mess used to be. Only then did the people at the shop realize that the "crazy" woman was an immortal and her "son" was actually her gourd (Zhao 1936, 47).

The lesson of this story is: before you made fun at people who appear to be crazy, consider the possibility that they might be immortals!

We have seen in this chapter that madness was not a newly recognized phenomenon in Qing China. At both the classical medical and popular levels there existed a rich body of literature that dealt with the illness in great detail. We see from the cases and stories presented here that while the afflicted persons and their families were sometimes at a loss as to the most appropriate treatment for the condition, they were nonetheless familiar with the realm of possibilities; although madness was a strange illness, it was not unfamiliar. We know also that families played a crucial role in the management of the insane, and that physicians, priests, and exorcists were only part of the larger health care system.

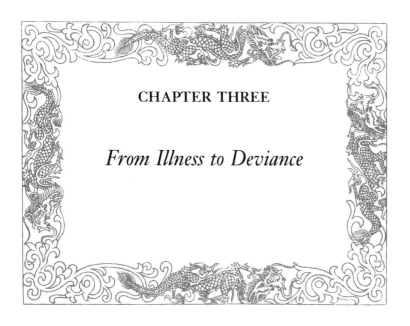

CHAPTER THREE

From Illness to Deviance

IN 1731, THE GOVERNOR-GENERAL of Sichuan submitted a memorial to the Yongzheng emperor in which he argued for the implementation of mandatory confinement of the insane. He was prompted to do so by a recent case of multiple homicide committed by an insane man. In his memorial, the governor-general presented the homicide as a symptom of a larger problem. He opined that unrestrained maniacs posed a threat to society and proposed that measures be taken to put them under tighter control. More specifically, he recommended mandatory registration and confinement. He himself had experimented briefly with a voluntary program in Sichuan, but because of the lack of legal sanctions, his scheme had been ignored by both citizens and local law enforcement officials.

The multiple homicide, he submitted, was a tragic consequence. Families could not be counted on to lock up their relatives voluntarily, because this seemed too cruel. Neighbors would not report instances of noncompliance, because they did not want to meddle in other people's business. District magistrates could not be relied on to enforce voluntary confinement, because they had no incentive to do so. And as long as the surveillance and control of maniacs did not figure in their annual evaluations (*kaocheng*), they would continue to ignore the problem (*Cheng'an zhiyi* 1755, 19:42a–42b).

The proposal for tighter control of insane persons residing in Sichuan was made at a most opportune time. The Yongzheng emperor had only recently taken a personal interest in Sichuan affairs and, particularly, the high level of unrest in the province. The crime problem in Sichuan was a legacy of the resettlement policy that was implemented at the beginning of the Qing dynasty to repopulate areas devastated by the uprisings and banditry of the late Ming period. Many of the early immigrants staked out huge acreages for reclamation, but because they could not cultivate them by themselves, they farmed out portions of their holdings to tenant farmers who, in turn, also sublet portions of the rented land to still other tenants. The exact size of the staked-out areas was more often than not left unrecorded, and the names of landowners were frequently not registered. After several decades of ad hoc arrangements, many of the actual cultivators had no idea who were their landlords, nor did the landlords know who were their tenants. Disputes over boundaries and rents grew more and more frequent, and rich and powerful families sometimes resorted to brute force to seize land from newer settlers, causing displacement and economic hardship. By the 1720s, it became clear to the government that the situation in Sichuan had become extremely volatile. According to Suzuki, the situation was further exacerbated because many of the later immigrants were victims of swindlers who had beguiled them with rags-to-riches tales about Sichuan. In their eagerness to seek new and greater fortunes, many small landholders sold their meager holdings to the swindlers in order to raise funds for travel to

Sichuan. Unfortunately, many of them found that they had arrived too late, and that the best they could hope for was to be tenant farmers. The government responded to the crisis by adopting a two-pronged approach. The immediate problem of poverty and discontent was addressed by a financial assistance plan, which, unlike earlier financial aid measures, was more a form of relief than incentive to migrate. At the same time, the whole question of unrestrained migration into Sichuan came under intense review and it was decided in 1728 that immigration to Sichuan should be tightly controlled. In 1729, some officials even proposed that free movement of people from one province to another should be curtailed, and that only those with resettlement permits could be allowed to emigrate. Furthermore, it was recommended that those found without any means of livelihood should be sent back to their native places. Vagrancy had become a serious problem in Sichuan because, by the Yongzheng period, poor and unemployed people constituted a large part of the immigrant population (Suzuki 1974, 155–57; Entenmann 1980, 40–44).

It is clear, then, that the central government was very concerned about the disruptive consequences of uncontrolled migration of people to Sichuan and had been searching for ways to cope with the problem. The political climate was favorable to any proposal that promised to restore and maintain order. Circumstantial evidence suggests that the mandatory registration-confinement proposal might be related to this general concern about Sichuan. The proposal was doubly attractive because it gave one explanation for incidents of violence in Sichuan by identifying the insane as a class of socially disruptive and dangerous people, and it offered a specific program for neutralizing this threat to public order and welfare. The governor-general's proposal would impress upon his superiors in Beijing that he was aware of the crime problem in Sichuan and that he was actively engaged in tackling it. In any case, the recommendation was approved by the Board of Punishments as well as the Yongzheng emperor. For good measure, it was decided that mandatory registration and confinement of the insane should be implemented throughout the empire (*Cheng'an zhiyi* 1755, 19:42a–42b).

The emperor's response to the proposal to register and confine the insane in Sichuan was typical of his approach to governance—he liked proposals that offered specific solutions to specific problems. For example, in 1724, during the second year of his reign, the emperor received a memorial from Governor Shi Wenzhuo of Henan that detailed very specific measures to deal with the deficit problem in Henan. According to Zelin:

> The emperor's reply to [Shi Wenzhuo's] memorial is very revealing. Unlike the noncommittal responses he made to officials who tried to bend the rules and continue the use of funds from the informal network, [Yongzheng's] rescript openly praised [Shi's] plan. The emperor told him that this memorial could not be compared with the vague mutterings in his previous memorials. [Yongzheng] pointed out that a high provincial official's duty lay precisely in this kind of thorough attention to fiscal matters. . . . Platitudes about morality and good government were not enough. (1984, 95)

No wonder the Sichuan scheme to deal with a potentially dangerous segment of the population found approval from the Yongzheng court. It showed the kind of attention to detail that the emperor demanded from his high provincial officials.

The Great Confinement

Mandatory registration and confinement meant, in effect, placing the insane under house arrest. Families with insane members were required to register them with their district magistrates or banner captains (*zuoling*), after which they were to be confined at home and kept under strict surveillance by family members as well as neighbors. Insane persons who did not have relatives to care for them were put in the joint custody of neighbors, clan elders, and local constables. As a goad for compliance with this order, the board made it known that the relatives and/or neighbors of insane persons who committed suicide or homicide would be held accountable and duly punished (eighty blows for suicide and one hundred blows for homicide). Mindful of the fact that magistrates and banner captains, too, needed incentives to take on the additional responsibility, the board warned that any suicide or homicide committed by the insane that could be attributed to the officials' own laxity would cost them part of their salary—three months' salary for suicide and twelve months' for homicide (*Cheng'an zhiyi* 1755, 19:42a–42b). This order was formally incorporated into the Qing Code as a substatute in 1740 (*Xing'an huilan* 1968, 2114; Nakamura 1973, 189).

In 1766 the Qing government amended the 1740 substatute in order to make more stringent the conditions of confinement. After registration, the insane could be turned over to their families for confinement at home only if the authorities were satisfied that their families had a place, such as a barred room, to keep them locked up at all times. Otherwise, they would have to be incarcerated in government jails, where common criminals were held. Those who did not have families to take care of them were also kept in jails. In keeping with the Confucian tradition of propriety which excluded women from prisons unless they had committed a capital offense, insane women were routinely discharged to the care of their families after registration. To ensure that home confinement was just as secure as incarceration, the government even provided locks and chains (*DXXA* 1908, Renming, 92a–93b; Nakamura 1973, 189–91). Like the earlier substatute, however, this law did not specify punishment for simple noncompliance. Presumably, as long as families managed to keep their sick relatives out of harm's way, they would not be prosecuted for their failure to comply with the laws. Such an omission would seem to invite noncompliance which could have undermined the effectiveness of the whole mandatory registration-and-confinement program.

For those whose families had complied with the laws, reintegration into society was permitted only after the registered person had been certified as completely well. To prevent fraudulent claims of recovery, the 1766 law required clan elders, the local constable, and *baojia* headmen to submit bonded statements which corroborated the family's claim and to pledge

their willingness to accept responsibility for the future conduct of the recovered registrant. Those confined in government jails, on the other hand, had to wait "several" years after
the disappearance of the recognized symptoms of madness before they could be released (*DXXA* 1908, Renming, 92a–93b;
Nakamura 1973, 189–91). This was probably because the government wanted to make sure their recovery was permanent
before allowing them to reenter society. Interestingly, although
China had such a long and sophisticated medical tradition,
and physicians had recourse to a rich corpus of medical literature regarding madness, there was no stipulation of any official
role for physicians in the certification process. The conspicuous absence of physician participation in this process drives
home the point that doctors were generally held in low esteem
in the Qing period (Smith 1983, 226). This was in marked
contrast to the situation in England, where trials involving insane offenders became, in the words of Roger Smith, "trials by
medicine" (1981b).

The substatute did not state clearly—as the 1731 circular
did—that insane persons should be registered with magistrates or banner captains. Instead, the rather ambiguous term
"supervising official" was used. For those officials who were
familiar with the legislative history of these two substatutes,
there was perhaps no doubt that "supervising official" meant
both magistrates and banner captains, and that mandatory
registration and confinement was applicable to both commoners and bannermen alike. However, it seems that the am-
biguity did cause some confusion among the less-informed
officials, so that in 1806, the Statutes Commission felt compelled to issue a memorandum to advise officials at all levels of
government that the mandatory registration-and-confinement
requirement did apply to bannermen and their bondservants
(*Xing'an huilan* 1968, 2127–28).

The registration-and-confinement scheme bore a striking
similarity to the Qing program for the control of repatriated
thieves. The duty of supervising the convicted thief was initially assigned to a relative, usually the father or elder brother,
who was held accountable for the conduct of his charge. Un-

derstandably, many families were reluctant to assume such an onerous responsibility, and the burden was later placed on the constable and *baojia* headmen. These local police agents were required not only to keep a vigilant watch over the paroled thieves but also to guarantee their good behavior (Chen 1975, 121–42).

Placing the insane under virtual house arrest or in prison, whether or not they had committed any crimes, was tantamount to labeling them "criminal deviants." The fact that local police agents were recruited into the registration-and-confinement program for the purpose of maintaining surveillance as well as to guarantee good behavior—just as they were required to do with repatriated thieves—further substantiates this interpretation.

Because there were no institutions of confinement other than prisons, the government was limited to putting the insane under virtual house arrest or in jail. This was in marked contrast to France and England, where *hôpitaux généraux*, poorhouses, and special hospitals such as Brideswell and Bethlem were established to accommodate (and in a sense, quarantine) all sorts of undesirables, including indigents, vagrants, and invalids as well as lunatics. According to Andrew Scull, the evolution in England of specialized institutions to house the deviant population was closely related to the growth of centralized monarchy in the sixteenth century. This resulted in a diminution of the role of the church in civil society which, in turn, affected the way the sick and homeless were cared for. Subordination of the church by the state forced an institutional approach to those who could not be integrated into the mainstream (see Scull 1979). These dynamics were not present in China, where the family was traditionally the care provider. Since the Chinese state did not view the family as a threat (in the way that the church was a threat to the state in England), there had been no impulse to diminish the role of the family in society and, consequently, no compelling reason for the state to establish hospitals or similar institutions to accommodate the sick and homeless. Thus, even during Qing times, when the government was most centralized, the notion that the state should "nationalize" such care was simply not in the collective mentality at all.

Nonetheless, mandatory registration-and-confinement was in many respects a legal innovation that violated Chinese tradition. In the first place, it contradicted the ancient principle of concealment whereby juniors in a family were forbidden by law to inform on their seniors. Secondly, it violated the paramount virtue of filial piety by forcing children to keep insane parents under lock and chain. The mandatory registration-and-confinement program, therefore, could have been conceived only by a government that was obsessed with social control. Xue Yunsheng, the noted late Qing legal scholar and Board of Punishments official, recognized the social implications of the mandatory registration-and-confinement substatutes. In his commentary on Qing laws, *Duli cunyi* (first published in 1905), he criticized the 1766 law for violating Chinese tradition as well as for "criminalizing" the insane:

> The right to conceal crimes committed by one's father or grandfather is legally sanctioned, and yet the children and grandchildren of an insane person are required by this substatute to inform the authorities of his condition and to keep him locked up [like a common criminal]. . . .
> The most ludicrous aspect of this law, however, is the requirement that those who [could not be accommodated at home] must be sent to prison and kept there. If we do not imprison criminals who committed minor offenses, why should we imprison the insane? To confine them for life [simply because of their condition] is tantamount to saying that insane people are by nature murderers. Can this be called rational?
> This law is a product of an [irrational] fear, stemming from a few isolated cases of homicide committed by insane persons, that all insane people are potential murderers. To involve all because of the action of one is [unconscionable as well as impracticable]. This law is meaningless. (Xue 1970, 860)

Xue was not exaggerating when he suggested that commitment was tantamount to long-term imprisonment. The following case supports his contention:

In 1845 Liu Chaoyuan, a native of Sichuan province, was

committed to prison at the request of his elder brother. Six months later, when the brother suddenly died, Liu's widowed mother sought his release, pleading that she was old and had no son to care for her. The governor-general of Sichuan, to whom the case was forwarded, was sympathetic and conveyed his support for her petition to the Board of Punishments. He made special note of the fact that Liu had not suffered a relapse during his confinement in prison and, more importantly, he had never committed any reprehensible act.

The Board of Punishments did not immediately approve the request. While conceding that there were legitimate reasons for Liu's release from prison—that Liu was the sole surviving son and that his mother was aged and needed someone to take care of her—the board noted that he had been confined for only slightly more than six months, well short of the "several years" stipulated by law. The board ordered the governor-general to ascertain the completeness of Liu's recovery, to assess his mother's ability to control him, and to look into the matter of having a barred room readied for Liu's confinement at home in case of a future relapse. Only after such precautionary measures had been taken could Liu be allowed to return home. Otherwise, he was to be kept in prison for several more years, after which his release would be deliberated again (*Xing'an huilan xupian* 1970, 2993–2995). Given the fact that Liu Chaoyuan was committed at his brother's request, which meant that the family residence did not have the requisite facilities to keep him confined at home in the first place, it is likely that his mother's petition for immediate release was not granted.

The cautious attitude of the Board of Punishments was by no means unjustified. There had been instances where prematurely released insane inmates later suffered relapses and created havoc. In 1826, for example, the Board of Punishments was asked to review the release request forwarded by the magistrate of Daxing on behalf of a prisoner's father. The insane inmate in question, Yang San, had a history of episodic madness. He had once before been briefly confined in a government jail, in compliance with the mandatory registration-and-confinement substatutes. He was released from his confinement when the local officials determined to their own satisfaction that he had recovered fully from his illness. In retrospect, this was an unwise decision, because Yang suffered a relapse and, under the influence of his illness, commandeered someone's donkey and rode it recklessly up and down the streets of his native town. He was apprehended by soldiers and sent to the yamen of the provincial commander-in-chief. He was later transferred to a jail supervised directly by the Board of Punishments, where he was examined and certified as genuinely insane. At that time, because his father testified that a room could not be set aside for his confinement at home, the board committed him to the county jail at Daxing, where he remained confined under the supervision of the magistrate. It was thus that Yang San was incarcerated again. Not long afterwards, his father petitioned the magistrate to have his son released from his imprisonment. The magistrate, after having Yang San examined, was satisfied that the prisoner had fully recovered from his illness, and was supportive of the father's request.

Not surprisingly, given Yang's history, the board was reluctant to set him free. They noted that his second confinement had lasted less than one year, well short of the "several years after recovery" requirement stipulated by the relevant substatutes. Such being the case, it was inappropriate to consider the question of his release. However, since it was his father who had initiated the petition, the magistrate should, as a gesture of courtesy, follow through with the request and ascertain from his father whether he was able to keep Yang under constant surveillance at home and whether, in the case of a relapse, he could provide a secure room where Yang could be locked up (*Xing'an huilan* 1968, 2113).

The prospect of lengthy confinement was made even more intolerable by the atrocious conditions in Chinese prisons (see Bodde 1969). Prisons were holding facilities where criminals awaiting the final outcome of the review process were kept. The "temporary" nature of incarceration fostered an official indifference to prison conditions. Prisoners often had to buy their own food and firewood from the warden, who relied on the sale of such items for his livelihood, since he was not paid by the government. Inmates whose families could not afford to bribe the warden or to buy them food suffered greatly. In fact, the mortality rate was so high that, according to one account, a morgue was considered to be a necessary adjunct (Gray 1878, 1:46–53).

The substatute did not specify how insane inmates should be treated. It is not clear, for instance, whether they were segregated from the rest of the prison population. However, available information on prison life in the Qing period suggests that single-occupant cells were nonexistent. One of Derk Bodde's sources, Fang Bao, estimated that there were fifty or more prisoners on his ward; another source, Harry Parkes, counted seventy-three. That prisoners were grouped together in large numbers was not unusual, for, as Bodde points out, "the incarceration of prisoners in large groups rather than in single or dual confinement is a good example of Chinese family- and group-mindedness" (Bodde 1969, 317).

If the insane inmates were not separated from the other prisoners, what measures might have been taken to safeguard them as well as their cell mates? Bodde's essay provides us with a clue:

> Occupants of the Board's prison slept crowded together on a low wooden bench which extended about eight feet out from one wall of the ward, sloping slightly toward this wall. Chains suspended from overhead beams were used to confine serious criminals by passing the short chain connecting their handcuffs through a link of the large hanging chain. . . . According to the statute, the number of chains to be worn by each chained prisoner differed according to the seriousness of his offense. (1969, 317–18)

Given that even those who were confined at home were required by law to be chained and fettered, it is likely that those who were incarcerated in government jails were chained as well. If such was the case, insane inmates were treated the same way as serious criminals. Not only was insanity criminalized, but those who had the misfortune of being committed to government jails for the duration of their illness probably were treated worse than common criminals. It does not require much imagination to conclude that mandatory registration-and-confinement was neither practical nor enforceable in family-oriented China.

The reader may recall that in 1731, when the governor-general of Sichuan recommended legal sanctions for registration and confinement, he noted the reluctance on the part of families to comply with his lockup order because it seemed too cruel to them. The substatutes of 1740 and 1766 actually did not go far enough to ensure universal compliance. In spite of the Qing penchant for spelling out precise penalties for every conceivable offense, there was no provision in either law for noncompliance. That is to say, as long as families managed to keep their sick relatives out of harm's way, they would not be prosecuted simply for failing to comply with the laws. And as long as lengthy incarceration in prison remained a distinct possibility, there was really no reason for the families voluntarily to submit to registration and confinement. Unfortunately, the decision to disregard the law and risk the consequences sometimes resulted in tragedy for the entire family. For example, in 1816, a man with a history of episodic madness went berserk, killing his parents, his wife, and a sister-in-law. His brother later testified that the family opted not to register him with the authorities because they were afraid that the officials might send him to prison (*Yuedong cheng'an chupian* 1882, 13:23a).

Local Resistance

It is impossible to provide statistical evidence to show that the mandatory registration-and-confinement program failed. However, a survey of all the relevant criminal cases concerning insane offenders reveals that the vast majority of the offenses were committed by those who had never been registered. Only a small fraction of the crimes were committed by those who suffered a relapse after release from confinement. In 1908 the government acknowledged the futility of enforcing an impractical law. It struck the registration-and-confinement substatutes from the revised Qing Code (*DXXA* 1908, Renming, 92a–93b).

For the program to succeed, it had to rely on the viability of the *baojia* system as an instrument of local control. However, as Kung-chuan Hsiao demonstrates, the system failed to live up to the expectations of the Qing emperors. According to Hsiao, it was confronted with almost insurmountable difficulties and obstacles in many aspects of its operation. Take, for example, the registration of households:

> In the first place, the method of registration prescribed by law proved difficult to execute. Each household . . . was required to have a [*menpai*], or door placard, on which the names of the members were to be written. The average villager seldom was able to fulfill this seemingly simple requirement; and the gentry often chose to sabotage the registration procedure altogether. Some officials tried to remedy the situation by simplifying the requirement. . . . There is no evidence that such measures removed the fundamental obstacle to registration: the general unwillingness to register. (1960, 75)

If the populace proved to be unwilling to comply with the general registration requirement, with its rather simple procedure which would not stigmatize any member of their households, it is not surprising that they would resist the idea of registering a family member as insane. More importantly, if the *baojia* headmen had difficulty in meeting their basic registration obligations, it would be unrealistic to expect them to play a significant role in the registration of insane persons in their units.

Another important function of the *baojia* system was police control, which would include surveillance and control of the insane. Supposedly, members of the *baojia* units had the legal obligation to report crimes, criminals, and other suspicious persons to their *baojia* heads. However, according to Hsiao:

> This requirement appears simple, but in practice it was not at all easy to fulfill. Crimes serious enough to merit government attention were seldom committed by timid men; on the con-

trary, they were likely to be the work of persons who had little respect for the lives and property of their fellow villagers. The average householder, knowing that the vengeance of such men was fearful and that whatever protection the government might offer was uncertain, far away, and slow to come, found it more prudent not to incur the wrath of desperadoes than to fulfill a legal obligation which the government often failed to exact. Keeping silence therefore was less risky than reporting what one knew. . . . Eventually villagers learned to practice the axiom: "Each sweeps the snow in front of his own door and pays no attention to the hoarfrost on another man's roof." (1960, 78)

When the government responded to the problem of nonreporting by implementing the system of joint pledge and mutual responsibility, in which neighbors were mutually responsible for the conduct of all, the measure backfired. The people evaded the burden of mutual responsibility with a conspiracy of silence (ibid., 79).

We can see, then, that one of the basic components of the mandatory registration-and-confinement program, the *baojia* system, was not up to the tasks that it was originally intended for. It was simply not capable of taking on new responsibilities such as the surveillance and control of insane persons in the local communities.

The Qing government also intended to use the clan organization as a means of rural control. Toward this end, in 1757, the government formally adopted a system which required the clans to elect from among their membership persons who would serve as *zuzheng* and who would, in that capacity, be responsible for investigating and reporting the good and bad elements of the clans. The hidden agenda was that by giving the clan a formal, legal status, the government could bring the entire clan organization directly under its control. At first glance, this seemed to be an ingenious move. After all, the family, and, by extension, the clan, made up the fabric of Chinese society; if the government could co-opt clan organization to serve its interests, the tentacles of imperial power could extend to the lowest reaches of society. However, the system contained a serious flaw. Hsiao sums it up very well:

In employing the clan to help strengthen its control over the countryside, the imperial government treated the kinship group more as a supplementary police organ than as a social body characterized (to borrow a phrase from the Sacred Edict) by the principle of "harmony and affection." In fact, the law which required the [*zuzheng*] to report lawbreakers among their own kinsfolk was in a sense contrary to this principle; it might even conflict with the Confucian idea that the root of human virtue lay in the sanctity of family relationships. Moreover . . . clans often preferred to have erring members dealt with by their own elders rather than hand them over to government officials. In making the [*zuzheng*] a virtual [*baojia*] agent, therefore, the [Qing] rulers did some violence both to the basic conception and natural propensities of the clan (1960:350).

The problem was compounded by the fact that the *zuzheng* and the traditional clan leader, *zuzhang*, were not necessarily the same person. When they were different individuals, the *zuzheng* was the official clan leader, chosen to meet the requirements of the government. On the other hand, the *zuzhang* was the unofficial leader, chosen by the clan members on their own accord and, by virtue of this fact, given more respect than the *zuzheng*. The *zuzheng*'s standing within his own clan was undermined because he was not its natural leader. Had the government stipulated that the traditional clan head should also be the police agent, the hold of the government over the clan organization might have been much stronger.

It is noteworthy that there was no mention of *zuzheng* in any of the mandatory registration-and-confinement directives and substatutes. Rather, it was the *zuzhang* who was assigned the responsibility of guaranteeing the conduct of his insane kinfolk. Could it be possible that the omission of *zuzheng* from the wording of the directives and substatutes was, in fact, a tacit acknowledgment by the lawmakers of the reality that the *zuzheng* system was not functional and therefore could not be trusted?

As it turned out, the *zuzhang* could not be trusted either. First of all, it was the "natural propensity" (to borrow Hsiao's expression) of the clans to take care of their problems internally. And if they were to "behave with generosity to kindred, in order to demonstrate harmony and affection," as they were exhorted to do by the Qing emperors, it was to be expected that they would care for their sick members privately and would not turn them over to the authorities for fear of condemning their kinfolk to imprisonment. Self-interest also militated against the clan leader's voluntary participation in the registration-and-confinement program. Once a person was registered with the authorities as insane, he or she immediately became the responsibility of the family, the clan, neighbors, the *baojia* apparatus, the local constable, and the district magistrate or banner captain. It was so much easier for everyone, including the clan leader, to feign ignorance than to accept the onerous assignment of watching over the duly-registered person. We find, once again, a conspiracy of silence.

Another weak link in the mandatory registration-and-confinement scheme was the district magistrate. Laws are only as effective as those who enforce them, and there is no evidence to show that the magistrates took very seriously the responsibility of controlling the insane in their administrative areas. Readers may recall that when the governor-general of Sichuan implemented his own scheme in the 1720s, he realized to his chagrin that his magistrates did very little to carry out his plan. And he understood correctly that as long as the control of insane persons was not a factor to be considered during the annual evaluation process (*kaocheng*), there was very little incentive for the overworked magistrates to pay attention to it. He spelled this out clearly in his 1731 memorial.

Although his proposal for mandatory registration-and-confinement became the basis for the 1731 circular and subsequent substatutes, his suggestion that the *kaocheng* process be made a part of the control program was not adopted by the central government. While magistrates were held accountable for the conduct of the insane persons living in their districts, they were disciplined and punished only if it could be established that they had been lax in their supervision of registered maniacs. The incentive was there for them *not* to encourage registration. As in the case of the *baojia* heads and clan leaders,

it was preferable to feign ignorance than to assume the onerous responsibility of supervising the conduct of the registrants.

Another source of local resistance, and one which perhaps
did not occur to the government at all, lay in popular conceptions of and attitudes toward madness. It was noted in Chapter
One that for the medical establishment of China, madness carried no stigma. The same could not be said of the common
people, especially those who believed in supernatural causes of
illness. Among the myriad popular explanations for madness,
perhaps the most damning was that of divine retribution, because it held the insane person morally responsible for his or
her condition. One can understand, therefore, reluctance on
the part of the family to admit that one of its members had
become mad. They themselves most likely would attribute the
madness to causes other than divine retribution, but because
they had no control over what other people might think about
their afflicted kin, there was a compelling reason for them
to hide the fact of the illness from others, including the
government.

Insanity and Criminal Responsibility

The transformation of madness from illness to criminal deviance generated the need to formulate new laws that specifically addressed crimes committed by the insane—the newly
recognized class of malefactors. As a result, Qing jurists were
compelled to broach an issue that had hitherto not been given
particular attention, that of criminal responsibility of the
insane.

The question of whether insane offenders should be punished forced officials in the eighteenth century to examine the
problem of criminal insanity. No elaborate exegesis on the subject was articulated at the time; however, a clue to their understanding can be found in the expression *fengfa wuzhi*, which
appeared frequently in trial records. *Fengfa wuzhi* may be
loosely translated as "a lack of awareness due to insanity." But
what did jurists mean by "lack of awareness" (*wuzhi*)? As far as
one can determine from the trial records, there was no rigid
interpretation of what constituted *wuzhi*. Much depended on

the judicial officials' idiosyncratic conceptions of insanity. The following robbery-murder serves as an example:

One day in 1757, a cattle trader named Zhou Shiliang asked his cousin, Zhou Shihong, to accompany a customer home in order to collect the balance of a bill. The next morning, having collected the amount, Zhou Shihong set off for his cousin's house with two sacks of money. Upon passing through a desolate, hilly area, Zhou was ambushed by an agitated young man, Wu Lin'er, who stabbed him about twenty times before fleeing with one of the sacks.

Part way home, Wu stashed part of the money next to a haystack, covering it with an armful of hay, before continuing home to his mother. At the sight of her blood-smeared, knife-wielding son, the horrified mother hurriedly yanked him into the house, out of the neighbors' view, where she stripped off his stained clothing. Wu seemed oblivious to his mother's frantic activity, but when she began to pull some money out of the sack he suddenly sprang up, snatched the money, and sprinted out of the house with it. Later that day, when his father, Wu Changhua, came home, his wife showed him the stained clothing and money sack. Picking up the sack, he noted the character "Zhou" on it and realized instantly that his son was in serious trouble; he had heard that a man called Zhou Shihong had been found robbed and murdered. Instead of going to the authorities, he decided to cover up for his son.

In the meantime, a neighbor, Wu Ruibi, discovered the hidden money and unwittingly set off a chain of events. First, on his way home with the windfall, he ran into Lin'er, who instantly recognized the money and demanded that Ruibi hand it over to him. Ruibi at first thought that the money probably belonged to Changhua, and was about to hand it over to Lin'er, when he remembered that the youth had a history of erratic behavior and thought that the money might not be safe with him; a better alternative was to keep the money for a while and then return it to Changhua at a later time. While Ruibi was thus vacillating, Lin'er continued to badger him, so much so that Ruibi finally decided that he had better take the money directly to Changhua before the youth had the chance to accuse him of theft. Changhua knew, of course, that the money was not his, but he had no choice but to accept it since refusing it would stir up suspicions. Nine days later, he developed a case of jitters and decided to return the money to Ruibi, who did not seem to mind at all. Eventually, rumors about the money and Lin'er's complicity reached the district magistrate. Lin'er was arrested and his father was ordered to come forward with the blood-stained clothing, murder weapon, and money sack.

Throughout the trial, Lin'er refused to cooperate with the authorities, maintaining stony silence even when tortured (judicial torture was permissible). Lin'er's behavior complicated matters for the magistrate. On the one hand, he was inclined to believe that Lin'er was mad because no sane person could possibly remain unmoved by torture. On the other hand, he doubted that Lin'er was insane because Lin'er would not have robbed Zhou if he were really mad. The magistrate finally convinced himself that the madness was real, and recommended that Lin'er be kept in prison until he had fully recovered. The magistrate's judgment was upheld by his superior, the governor, who forwarded the case to the Board of Punishments for review.

The Board of Punishments was not convinced that Wu Lin'er was insane, and a retrial was ordered. Specifically, the board wanted the governor to review the following aspects of the case: (1) the robbery—board officials wondered if the robbery demonstrated that Lin'er was not really mad, because in their mind, an insane person simply could not know the love of money; (2) the matter of the hidden money—the board doubted that an insane person would have the wit to hide his loot; (3) Lin'er's instant recognition of his hidden loot; (4) his calm disposition when his mother took off his clothes—the board felt that an insane person under similar circumstances would have put up a struggle.

The retrial was essentially an exercise on the part of the provincial officials to reconfirm their original judgment, and they managed to do so quite ingeniously. Regarding Lin'er's "love of money," the governor replied that if the accused really loved money, he would have taken *all* that Zhou Shihong had with him at the time of the ambush, not just a fraction of it. Moreover, the governor pointed out, Lin'er lost most of the loot. Such carelessness about money could only mean that he did not know its value.

As for the part of the loot found by Wu Ruibi, the governor reported that new information provided by Ruibi during the retrial revealed that the money had actually been abandoned by Lin'er. According to the governor, Ruibi volunteered the information that it was his custom to arrange armfuls of hay to perch at an angle atop his haystacks to serve as a kind of rain shelter. Ruibi himself offered the speculation that Lin'er perhaps had absentmindedly thrown the money into one of his haystacks, and that the money subsequently slid to the ground, taking with it some of the precariously perched hay, which fell on top of the money. Although the governor conceded that Ruibi's hypothesis was a bit too farfetched to be valid, he argued that if Lin'er had really wanted to hide the money, he would have found a safer place for it, and certainly not near a haystack where it could be discovered easily. The governor also submitted that if Lin'er knew enough to hide his loot, he would certainly have hidden the murder weapon as well, but in fact he flaunted it all the way home.

Concerning Lin'er's ability to recognize his loot, the governor pointed out that a normal person would have known better than to claim the money, since it was incriminating evidence. Lin'er's fuss over the money made it even more apparent that he was not aware of what he was doing or what he had done. As for Lin'er's alleged calm disposition when his mother took off his clothes, the governor admitted that in the rush to meet his deadline during the first trial, not enough attention was given to this aspect of the case. He reported that during the retrial, Lin'er's mother admitted that he did put up quite a fight and that she actually had to wrestle with him. We will never know whether the new information submitted by the governor in his second report was factual or fabricated to save his face, but the Board of Punishments evidently was satisfied with it and so his original judgment was upheld (*Cheng'an xin-pian* 1763, 9:14a–19a).

It is clear from the case presented above that the crux of the jurists' judgment was their conclusion that Wu Lin'er lacked the capacity to know what he was doing. For centuries, it was the accepted doctrine in Chinese law that inadvertent offenders should be granted clemency. B. E. McKnight points out that this legal tradition can be traced as far back as the founding of the Western Zhou dynasty (ca. 1027 B.C.). The Zhou founder was reported to have told his brother that justice meant strict punishment for deliberate malefactors, however minor the transgression, but full and complete pardon for inadvertent offenders, regardless of the severity of the crime (McKnight 1981, 2). We can see that criminal intent (mens rea) was established as an important factor in the determination of criminal responsibility very early in Chinese history. This legal tradition, in the end, informed and helped decide for Qing jurists the question of criminal responsibility of the insane. So it was that in 1766, the Board of Punishments made the following unequivocal statement: "Insane persons lack the capacity to reason and are not conscious of their actions. Therefore, it is difficult to assign any guilt to insane criminals. We must pardon inadvertent transgressions, however grave they might be" (*Dingli huipian* 1762–1883, 13:73a–73b). As we shall see in Chapter Four, this legal position was challenged over and over again with the result that in addition to mens rea, other considerations were also taken into account in determining the degree of criminal responsibility.

Another clue to the Qing understanding of criminal insanity is the formula-sentence, "So-and-so, because of insanity, killing so-and-so" (*yin feng sha ren*), which appeared in almost all reports on homicide committed by insane persons. This suggests that Qing jurists believed that violent acts committed by the insane were a product of their illness, which meant they were unable to control themselves and therefore should not be regarded as wilfull perpetrators.

The Qing formulations *fengfa wuzhi* and *yin feng sha ren* are similar in some respects to the reasonings behind the land-mark M'Naghten Rule (1843). In 1843, Daniel M'Naghten fired a shot at Drummond, private secretary to British Prime Minister Sir Robert Peel, mistaking him for the prime minister. Drummond died of his wounds five days later. M'Naghten was arrested and brought to trial, and his defense was brilliantly handled by Alexander Cockburn, who subsequently in his illustrious career became lord chief justice. One of Cockburn's tactical difficulties was that M'Naghten did not look like the stereotypical madman; in order to address this he resorted to the new conceptions on criminal insanity that were being articulated by some psychiatrists, most notably the American Isaac Ray. In essence, Ray maintained that then-current criteria for determining sanity, such as knowledge of the nature of the act and the ability to know right from wrong, were much too narrow. His point was that some genuinely insane individuals would not appear so to the untrained eye. Cockburn also made good use of Ray's observation that insanity had become a more common disease than people realized. However, his strategic dilemmas remained formidable. Nigel Walker summed up the situation:

> [Cockburn] had to establish not merely that partial insanity was within the law's interpretation of insanity, and that M'Naghten was partially insane; but also that his partial insanity in some way excused him. The latter proposition would have been less difficult to establish if it had been possible to argue that the accused had been so affected as to be unaware of what he was doing, or its consequences; but this was ruled out by the evidence. Another line of argument would have been that he had been so affected as to be unable to distinguish between right and wrong in general; but this too Cockburn never attempted to assert, probably because he felt that the rationality of most of his client's conduct made it implausible.
>
> If, on the other hand, he had argued that the nature of M'Naghten's delusion, while not rendering him generally incapable of telling right from wrong, had made him feel justified in this particular act, he risked two rejoinders. One was that this was not sufficient to satisfy at least some judges, who demanded a *general* incapacity to tell right from wrong. Another

was that even if his delusion had been the truth, M'Naghten would not have been acting in self-defence, under physical provocation or under duress of the kind which the law of God or man recognized as excusing homicide. The latter argument would of course have been fallacious, since if we assume that his delusion was true, and that it was M'Naghten's moral sense that was at issue, what mattered was not whether his act was justifiable in the eyes of God or man, but whether it was justifiable in M'Naghten's belief; if so, his partial insanity could have been held to prevent him from knowing whether this particular act was right or wrong. But these points would clearly have been risky ones to argue even before so sophisticated a bench, and Cockburn wisely did not do so.

What Cockburn did argue was that the prisoner's insanity "takes away from him all power of self-control." . . . At the end of his speech, when everyone's attention must have been flagging more than a little, he came as near as he dared to a summary of his argument: "I trust that I have satisfied you by these authorities that the disease of partial insanity can exist—that it can lead to a partial or total aberration of the moral senses and affections, which may render the wretched patient incapable of resisting the delusion, and lead him to commit crimes for which morally he cannot be held responsible."

The jury took very little time to render a special verdict, and M'Naghten was removed to Bethlem Hospital (1967–73, 93–94).

Not surprisingly, the verdict created an uproar. A few months later, the judges appeared before the House of Lords to explain the verdict and their interpretation of the law. The result of this public debate was the formulation of what came to be known as the M'Naghten Rule. To satisfy this test of criminal insanity, "the accused must either have been deprived of awareness of what he was doing or have been deprived of awareness that what he was doing was wrong; and it must have been a defect of reason, arising from the disease of the mind, and not mere ignorance, mistake, or perversity of opinion, which deprived him of this awareness" (ibid., 1967–73, 100).

Another tradition that can be traced back to the Western Zhou period was the principle of *sanshe* (three pardonables), which assigned diminished responsibility to offenders who were very young, very old, or mentally incompetent (*chunyu*). Later, in about A.D. 100, Chen Jong, a high-ranking court official, expanded the *chunyu* category to include insanity when he proposed to the emperor that "when a wildly insane and transformed person kills people he should be enabled to be sentenced to the decreased extreme penalty" (Hulsewé 1955, 301; Chiu 1981, 78). This tradition was continued and further elaborated in the Tang Code, which specified that lighter sentences be handed down to those who suffered from "incurable diseases" and those who suffered from "serious illnesses," a designation that included insanity (Nakamura 1973, 183–85; Bünger 1950, 1–9). Later on, when the government became reluctant to acquit insane murderers, the doctrine of diminished responsibility helped to ensure reduced punishment for these homicides.

It is important to note that Qing officials made a definite distinction between violent acts that were caused by insanity and those that, in their opinion, could only have been products of debasement. The following case supports this observation:

In 1762 Fei Bingre, a native of Taoyuan district in Jiangsu province, was charged with causing the deaths of seven members of his household. Fei was not an ordinary citizen. He was a member of the local gentry, and had served for a period of time as the *ruxue* (director of studies) of Taoyuan.

Fei Bingre had, over the years, married a total of five times and was widowed four times. His first wife hanged herself in 1743 because she could not tolerate his constant verbal abuse. His second wife drowned herself a year later after being hit in the mouth by Fei. Four years later, his third wife hanged herself because she could not endure living with him. After his fourth wife died—of natural causes—Fei married again, to a woman whose maiden name was Wang.

This Chinese Bluebeard had also taken four concubines and abused all of them. He beat one to death because he was unhappy with the way she managed the household finances. After killing her, he ordered two of his servants to wrap the body in a coarse rush mat and junk the remains in a common burial dump. He sent another concubine home to her parents, after subjecting her to repeated brutalization. A third concubine did not fare any better. Once, because she failed to prepare dinner to his satisfaction, he punished her by first battering her with a club and then searing her genitals with a red-hot prong. When she died of complications from the burns, he had her buried in a lot behind the house. He was equally cruel toward the fourth concubine, woman Gu. More than once, under the influence of alcohol, he responded to her rejections of his sexual demands by stabbing her with a knife, and during the winter of 1733, he cut off her right earlobe for no reason other than that he did not find the meal she had prepared for him to his liking. That same winter, he carved a piece of flesh from her back, barbecued it over a fire, and downed it himself with some rice wine, all because he found the woman's behavior toward him disagreeable.

In 1760, upon returning from a trip outside Taoyuan, Fei summoned woman Gu to the district seat to spend the night with him. When she showed up late, he forced her into a spread-eagle position and seared her genitals with a hot prong. When Gu's maid came to her mistress' rescue, she suffered burns on her face. Fei's victims were not limited to his wives and concubines. It was discovered later that he frequently abused his servants as well. In 1751 alone, he beat two of them to death and had their bodies abandoned in a common burial dump.

The atrocities described above were not revealed to the authorities until 1761. According to the report submitted by the provincial officials, Fei's private quarters were off limits to his servants and no one was allowed to enter without permission, so there were no eyewitnesses to his cruel deeds. As for his neighbors, they lived too far away to be certain that something was amiss, and they dared not go to the authorities without definite evidence, because unsubstantiated accusation was a punishable offense. No doubt Fei's status as a member of the local gentry also helped discourage his neighbors from bringing charges against him.

The opportunity to inform on Fei came in 1761, when the prefect of Huainan made an informal visit to Taoyuan. Since such visits were undertaken expressly to solicit information about wrongdoings in a particular area, informants were not required to provide ironclad proof to substantiate their suspicions. One such informant tipped off the prefect about Fei, who was arrested several months later. He confessed readily to the charges and the governor of Jiangsu sentenced him to death by "immediate" strangulation, the punishment prescribed by the substatute governing the crime of killing two junior members of a household. (See Chapter Four for explanation of different death penalties.)

When the case reached the capital for joint review by the Board of Punishments, the Court of Revision, and the Censorate, the governor's judgment was found to be too lenient. The metropolitan officials ruled:

> This perverted and evil man, Fei Bingre, had blatantly violated the laws of the land. He abused his wives, concubines, and servants, and caused the deaths of seven of them. Furthermore, his behavior toward the concubine Gu was especially heinous. Depraved persons such as he are completely beyond the normal order of things (changli zhiwai).
>
> The sentence recommended by the governor is really too light for such a serious offense. [But how shall we see to it that he gets the punishment that he deserves]? If we simply overturn the governor's ruling and send the case back to him for retrial, it will take far too much time. . . . We recommend therefore that Fei Bingre be sentenced according to another substatute, one that permits us to behead him as soon as possible. We believe that the substatute governing the punishment of "baresticks" serves this purpose very well.

The reviewers' recommendation was approved by the Qianlong emperor, and Fei Bingre was beheaded, without further ado, at the provincial seat of Jiangsu (Cheng'an xinpian 1763, 8:24a–26b). ("Baresticks" refers to ruffians who wielded sticks and swords to intimidate people.)

It is noteworthy that at no point did anyone entertain the idea that Fei was insane. He was variously labelled "brutal," "perverted," "cruel," "evil," and "depraved," but not "insane." Their condemnation of Fei as a person "beyond the normal order of things," and the conspicuous exclusion of insanity as a probable cause of his perverse deeds suggest that the Qing officials believed that the atrocities committed by Fei could only have been the work of one who had lost his humanity, not his sanity.

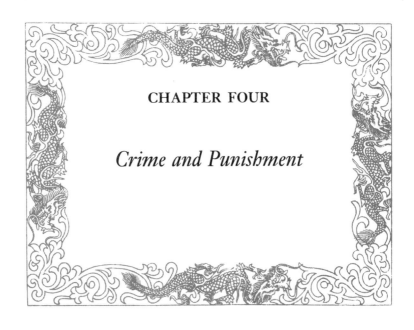

CHAPTER FOUR

Crime and Punishment

Abominations

ONE DAY IN 1775, Jin Mouming, the owner of a teahouse in Anqing, the capital of Anhui province, received a small parcel and a letter from a former neighbor who had moved to Jiangxi. Jin noticed the words *Kunzhi yuannian* (first year of the Kunzhi era), on the envelope and immediately realized their subversive implication. A new reign name was coined only upon the ascension to the throne of a new emperor; to suggest the beginning of a new era was tantamount to declaring the death of the reigning monarch, Qianlong. Fearing implication in a treasonous plot, Jin hurriedly delivered both the letter and the parcel to his district magistrate. The magistrate also recognized the sinister meaning of the scribbled words, and forwarded both items to Fei Congxi, the governor of Anhui.

Governor Fei immediately conducted a preliminary investigation of the incident and soon ascertained several pertinent facts. The sender of the letter, Wang Zuoliang, alias Wang Kunzhi, had become mad rather suddenly some time during the previous year and was escorted shortly afterwards from Anqing to his native Jiangxi by his elder brother. The letter he sent Jin consisted of four sheets of paper, on which a number of "obstinate" phrases and some thirteen names were scribbled. The contents of the parcel were rather bizarre—there were some pieces of religious paraphernalia along with a couple of pebbles.

Governor Fei sent an urgent request to his counterpart in Jiangxi, seeking extradiction of the Wang brothers to Anhui. He also asked the governor of Jiangxi to help him locate and arrest the thirteen persons whose names were listed in Wang's letter. He then rushed a report to the Qianlong emperor. The emperor was extremely displeased with Fei's handling of the incident and was particularly critical of Fei's lack of sound judgment. The proposed extradition of the Wang brothers and other material witnesses from Jiangxi to Anhui was, in his opinion, supremely foolish, for something untoward might happen to any one of them en route and thus undermine the government's efforts to get to the bottom of the matter. Also, Fei had failed to recognize the importance of the messenger who delivered the letter and parcel to Jin Mouming; after all, he might have been a key material witness. Equally inexplicable, in the emperor's opinion, was Fei's treatment of Jin, who was detained in prison although he had not violated any laws. In compensation for this maltreatment, the emperor ordered Fei to pay Jin a sum of money, not out of the government's account, but Fei's personal funds!

The Qianlong emperor then issued a set of instructions to Hai Cheng, the governor of Jiangxi. Wang Zuoliang and his brother, as well as all the material witnesses, should be detained in Jiangxi. Under no circumstances were they to be extradited to Anhui. Governor Hai was to take over the investigation and was to check thoroughly all aspects of the case, particularly one of Wang's cryptic notes, scribbled on a piece of religious paraphernalia, which accused a certain financial commissioner named Fei of being laggardly in the performance of his duties. The Qianlong emperor wanted to know if this was Fei Congxi.

At the same time the imperial orders were being sent to Jiangxi, the emperor received word from Hai that he had already decided to detain all the key witnesses in Jiangxi, and that he had begun interrogating them. The emperor was so pleased with Hai's initiative that he even sent a copy of Hai's memorial to Fei Congxi, for the latter's edification. Shortly afterwards, a second memorial from Hai reached Beijing, detailing the results of his investigation.

Hai confirmed Fei's earlier report that Wang had suddenly become insane and that his elder brother had taken him home to Jiangxi soon afterwards. Hai reported that about two months before, Wang had somehow managed to escape from his barred room at home. He found his way to a transportation company, where he entrusted his letter and parcel to the boat hand who delivered them to Jin. Hai was certain that Wang did not fake his madness. Not only did his neighbors and relatives all attest to the fact, but his erratic behavior during the interrogations also convinced the governor that the illness was genuine.

In spite of Wang's incoherence, Hai did manage to extract some pertinent information from him. He concluded that Wang was not a member of a heretical religious sect and thus was not a part of any organized rebellious movement. His religious scribblings were, in fact, quite harmless, and were in no way written to extort money from people (as were the products of religious charlatans). He seemed to have acted alone, and the thirteen people on his list were not in any way involved in the incident, nor did Wang have any intention of implicating them in a treasonous plot. Also, his accusations about the financial commissioner named Fei were nonsense.

Hai recommended the sentence of *lingchi* (death by slicing) for Wang Zuoliang. Although he did not doubt that Wang was insane, he would not allow the illness to be a mitigating factor in this case because the custom of treating inadvertent offenders with clemency was not applicable to heinous crimes. Inventing a new reign name was a treasonous act, thus there could not be any room for leniency. Hai also found Wang's elder brother culpable, for he should have been more vigilant in his watch over his sick brother. He therefore deserved the sentence of immediate decapitation. The emperor approved Wang Zuoliang's sentence, but he reduced the brother's by one degree to decapitation after the assizes (*Qianlong shilu* 1964, 14397–98; 14415; 14459).

Qianlong's active involvement in the case was not surprising. It is significant that the incident took shape almost on the heels of the Wang Lun Uprising of 1774. Although the millenarian rebellion in Shandong lasted only one month, and the central government was able to deal with it successfully, it was a harbinger of more ominous challenges that would plague the Qing for the remainder of the eighteenth and most of the nineteenth century. More immediately, it shocked the Qianlong emperor immensely to find this sectarian challenge to his authority in the heart of his empire, and it angered him even more to know that its suppression took a full month (Naquin 1981, xiv–xv). Thus, when news about the Wang Zuoliang incident reached the emperor in 1775, and circumstantial evidence at first indicated sectarian inspiration, it was to be expected that he would engage himself actively in efforts to get to the bottom of the matter as soon as possible.

The uncompromising position held by the government toward Wang was not unusual in the Chinese legal tradition. The Qing Code, following precedent set by earlier codes, specified the punishment of *lingchi* for offenses known as the Ten Abominations (*shi'e*): rebellion, disloyalty to the imperial house, desertion of duty, parricide, mass murder, sacrilege, lack of filial piety, initiation of discord within the family, insubordination to officials, and incest (Sprenkel 1977, 82; Bodde and Morris 1973, 93, 286). Severe punishment was deemed necessary because, as E. Balazs points out in his treatise on Sui law, the essence of all ten crimes was disobedience to authority (Sprenkel 1977, 82). Because treason, being the most serious challenge to the highest of all authorities, was considered the most heinous, the Qing Code provided the following punishments: *lingchi* for the principal offender (whether he actually committed or merely planned to commit treason); decapitation for the offender's father, grandfather, sons, grandsons, brothers, brothers' sons, paternal uncles, and others living with him in the same household; and slavery in the families of meritorious ministers for any of the above who are aged fifteen or less, as well as for the offender's mother, unmarried sisters and daughters, wife, and concubine(s), and wives and concubines of his sons (Bodde and Morris 1973, 286).

That Wang Zuoliang was unquestionably mad and therefore harbored no criminal intent did not make any difference in this case. Indeed, it is possible that the government recognized that Wang's undisputed illness made him an even better example (Governor Hai's statement hinted strongly at this possibility). The government's uncompromising stance served notice to all that treason was such a heinous crime that not even madness could be accepted as a mitigating factor in the determination of punishment.

Second only to the ruler-subject relationship in the Confucian scheme of the Three Bonds was that between father and son. We find that as was the case with treason, not even madness was accepted as a mitigating factor for the crime of parricide. In 1822, for example, a man killed his father during a fit of madness. He was killed on the spot by his mother, but neither his death nor his illness tempered the wrath of the Qing officials. They sentenced him, posthumously, to death by *lingchi*. His body was sliced up in public, for all to see (*XBJC* 1834, 21:6a–6b).

In the following year, 1823, the Board of Punishments again was faced with a case of parricide committed by an insane man. The board responded to this case with such vehemence that it was clear that the son's illness was regarded as only incidental. Reacting as though there had been an epidemic of parricide, the board sought permission from the Daoguang emperor to allow summary trial of insane parricides, so that the criminals could be executed without undue delay. The Daoguang emperor readily approved their request.

According to the circular that was sent out to judicial officials throughout the empire, criminals found guilty of killing their parents or grandparents during an affray should be executed without undue delay. No clemency would be shown toward the insane in these cases. At the time of sentencing, the governor would invoke the special procedure *gongqing wangming* (literally, "respectfully request royal authority"), which in effect empowered the governor to be the final arbiter in the case. This procedure ensured prompt execution of the death sentence, bypassing the usual, and time-consuming, reviews by the Board of Punishments and the emperor. As the circular pointed out, the abbreviated process guaranteed the government the opportunity to punish the criminal while he or she was still alive (*Xing'an huilan* 1968, 2763–64).

Why the Qing government chose to formulate such a harsh policy regarding insane parricides at this time, during the third year of the Daoguang reign, is a puzzle that begs solution. Perhaps a closer examination of the political climate of the mid-Qing period will yield some clues. When the Daoguang emperor ascended the throne in 1821, he inherited a host of problems. For example, the dynasty had been buffeted by a series of sectarian uprisings, the most famous (and perhaps the most threatening) of which was the White Lotus sect–inspired Eight Trigrams Rebellion of 1813. These uprisings were dangerous not only because of their violent nature, but because the ideology that informed them offered their followers an alternative to state-sponsored Neo-Confucianism. Susan Naquin sums it up very well:

> In the eighteenth century, the idea was widespread and deeply rooted that the one and only path to respect within Chinese society was through education in the Confucian Classics (validated by examination) and service in state bureaucracy. Thus, for those who shared the basic assumptions of the elite but found its institutional dominance suffocating or unsatisfying, White Lotus ideas and organization could be an alternative. The ways in which White Lotus sects mimicked the Neo-Confucian orthodoxy (with their own elites, classical texts, and historical vision) similarly indicates that no matter how slight their appeal, these sects both shared values with and considered

themselves the rivals of the elite. The fact that the authorities branded these sects as illegal and heterodox and prosecuted them out of all proportion to their popularity indicates that the [Qing] elite recognized competition when they saw it. (1981, 161)

The rush to judgment in 1823 seems to have been closely related to the sectarian challenge to Neo-Confucian orthodoxy. At the heart of the Confucian ethical system was the virtue of filial piety. In the opinion of Confucian moralists, children had to be filial toward their parents because they owed their very existence to them. This profound debt was further compounded by the years of selfless nurture provided them by their parents. Beginning with the Han Code, each successive dynastic code contained provisions that specified severe punishment for those found guilty of unfilial behavior, and beginning with the Northern Qi dynasty (550–577) impiety was listed as one of the Ten Abominations. Because of the centrality of filial piety in Confucian morality, and because of the close identification of Neo-Confucian orthodoxy with the Qing state, it was only to be expected that the government would continue the tradition of meting out the harshest punishment for unfilial conduct.

The decision reached in 1823 to ensure that insane parricides would live to suffer excruciatingly painful deaths by slicing had profound symbolic meaning. It signaled to members of the gentry class, whose continued cooperation and support were crucial to the survival of the dynasty, that the state remained a strong sponsor of Neo-Confucianism, so much so that it would not consider accepting insanity as a mitigating condition in the heinous crime of parricide. It also served notice to the deviant population that challenges to Neo-Confucian orthodoxy would not be tolerated. Indeed, when heterodox undercurrents threatened to pull under constituted authority, the Qing state—being the very embodiment of orthodox Confucian values—had no choice but to assert these values with a vengeance. Thus, as with treason, the need to defend orthodoxy rendered secondary the ancient doctrine of mens rea. In both treason and parricide cases, insanity was used by the government to make a stronger case for itself.

Treason and parricide were the two exceptions to the general principle of granting clemency to insane criminals. Sometimes this principle was challenged by officials who were genuinely concerned about the threat posed to society by insane persons who had proven themselves to be dangerous; others were wary of the possibility of hardened criminals exploiting the system by masquerading as madmen. Increasingly, these officials saw the need to strike a balance between the traditional sense of justice and their responsibility to protect society from criminal and dangerous elements. As will be shown in the following sections, the attainment of this balance was their Holy Grail.

Homicide in Qing Law

The substatutes formulated during the Qing period to deal with criminal acts committed by the insane were all homicide laws. Indeed, the subject of homicide in Qing criminal law is vast; the word *sha* ("to kill") itself was extremely comprehensive. Any act that, directly or indirectly, caused the death of another person was considered an act of homicide in traditional Chinese law. The Qing Code, in its treatment of the subject, differentiated well over twenty varieties of homicide. However, it is possible to group the myriad kinds of killing into six major categories: *mousha* (premeditated murder); *gusha* (homicide by instant design, intentional but not premeditated); *dousha* (homicide committed during an affray); *xisha* (killing during sport or horseplay); *wusha* (mistaken homicide, defined as killing an innocent bystander or a victim of mistaken identity; *guoshisha* (homicide by happenstance or accidental homicide). For a homicide to be considered *guoshisha*, it had to fit the requirement that "the use of eyes or ears could not have avoided the accident, and no care or thoughtfulness could have prevented it." Within these categories a distinction was also made between single and multiple homicides. The laws governing *xisha*, *wusha*, and *guoshisha* constituted a discrete group within the homicide section in the Qing Code. It was within this group that the substatutes concerning homicides committed by insane criminals were listed. There also were myriad death penalties to match crimes punishable by death. The most severe penalty was *lingchi*, just below which in degree of severity was decapitation, followed by strangulation. Both decapitation and strangulation were further classified as either "immediate" or "after the assizes." "Immediate" strangulation or decapitation meant that the sentence would be carried out as soon as the case had been reviewed and the penalty affirmed by the judicial authorities in Beijing. The execution of the sentence was almost certain. "After the assizes" meant that the sentence would be reconsidered at the Autumn Assizes in Beijing (Bodde and Morris 1973, 92–93).

The Insane Murderer: Single Homicide

The initial responses of the Qing government to violent acts committed by the insane tended toward leniency, but in 1669 it decided to exact a fine of sorts from insane murderers. The fine, which amounted to 12.42 taels of silver, was to be turned over to the victim's family as a kind of burial compensation. This initiative placed insane killers in the same penalty category as those who committed homicide as a result of negligence or accident. In 1725 this policy gained the formal status of substatute (Nakamura 1973, 190). The following case deliberated by the Board of Punishments in 1735 illustrates the law in action:

The governor-general of Zhili reported that Chong Fa, a native of Wei district, because of insanity fatally wounded his neighbor. The two men lived in the same compound, sharing a common courtyard, and got along well in the past. Chong had become insane a number of years earlier, but appeared to have recovered. In the autumn of 1734, however, he grew increasingly worried about the poor yield of his crops and was particularly concerned that he might not be able to meet his financial obligations. His anxiety eventually led to a relapse. His mother and wife confined him in a room in their house, but they failed to secure the door with a lock.

Several days into his confinement, he woke up one morning in a great state of agitation. He broke out of the room and, waving a wooden club, declared that he intended to slaughter the entire village. His neighbor Wei Bao heard the commotion and was about to lock the door to his own room when Chong burst in and began to bludgeon him with the club. Wei collapsed onto the floor. Having witnessed the horrifying scene, Chong's wife cried out for help. Several neighbors, along with Wei's wife, rushed to the room but it was too late. Wei had already died. Chong was apprehended and brought to trial.

By the time of his trial, Chong had already regained his senses. Nonetheless, the governor-general of Zhili was satisfied that he was insane at the time of the murder. He ruled that it was therefore inappropriate to sentence him to death, and instead invoked the single-homicide substatute of 1725, ordering Chong to pay Wei's widow 12.42 taels of silver to be used as funeral money.

At the same time, the governor-general held Chong Fa's mother, neighbors Chong Geng and Chong Youshi, *bao* unit headman Hou Guofu, and *jia* unit headman Zhang Jiuming accountable for his homicidal outburst. In his opinion, they were reprehensible because, in spite of their knowledge of Chong Fa's illness, they had failed to take proper action. They did not report him to the authorities, as they were required to do by the mandatory registration-and-confinement edict of 1731. Thus, it was their conspiracy of silence that led to the tragic killing. Chong Geng, Chong Youshi, and Zhang Jiuming were given the statutory sentence of one hundred blows with heavy bamboo. Chong Fa's mother, because she was a woman, was allowed to redeem her corporal punishment with money. As for Chong Fa himself, the governor-general recommended that he be incarcerated for a year or so, after which time, if he showed no signs of relapse, he could be returned to the custody of his family and neighbors. The judgment was upheld by the Board of Punishments (*Cheng'an zhiyi* 1755, 19:43a–43b).

This illustrates a problem left unresolved by the substatute of 1725: What other action needed to be taken after the burial compensation of 12.42 taels of silver had been made? Should the insane slayers be simply set free and left to their own devices? This would seem imprudent in light of the fact that they had already proven themselves to be a threat to public safety. The governor-general's innovative solution was to apply a provision of the 1731 mandatory registration-and-confinement law to the case and order imprisonment for at least one year. It was such a reasonable approach that the Board of Punishments formalized it in 1754 by incorporating it in a new substatute. Henceforth, insane killers would be required to remain in prison one year *beyond* the complete disappearance of all symptoms of madness. Officials soon realized, however, that it was almost impossible to determine accurately if a prisoner had completely recovered from insanity; they now appreciated the episodic nature of the illness, a point already noted in medical treatises. There did not seem to be any satisfactory guarantee that a released prisoner would not suffer a relapse and kill again. As a result of these uncertainties, in 1762 a new law was enacted that stipulated life imprisonment for insane murderers (*Xing'an huilan* 1968, 2114).

The primary concern that informed the substatutes of 1754 and 1762 was public safety. As a result of this concern Qing jurists decided that the ancient principle of clemency due inadvertent offenders could not be safely applied to insane criminals. Thus even though they continued to absolve insane murderers of criminal culpability, they could no longer set them free. This new position was remarkably similar to that arrived at in 1800 as a result of the landmark Hadfield case in England. That year, a man by the name of Hadfield fired a pistol at King George III, missing him by only inches. Hadfield was arrested and brought to trial; his lawyer was the famous John Erskine. After presenting a long series of witnesses who substantiated Hadfield's claim of insanity, Erskine urged the jury to return a verdict of acquittal. He softened their potential resistance (after all, Hadfield had almost killed their king) with the following presentation:

. . . the prisoner, *for his own sake, and for the sake of society at large* [italics mine], must not be discharged; for this is a case which concerns every man of every station, from the king upon the throne to the beggar at the gate; people of both sexes and of all ages may, in an unfortunate frantic hour, fall a sacrifice to this man, who is not under the guidance of sound reason; and therefore it is absolutely necessary for the safety of society that he should be properly disposed of, all mercy and humanity being shown to this most unfortunate creature. . . . (Walker 1967:78)

Erskine proved to be very persuasive. The jury returned a verdict of "not guilty" and Hadfield was eventually committed to Bethlem.

Nigel Walker provides a succinct analysis of the Hadfield case which is also instructive for our understanding the Qing experience:

It was acquittal in name only, for it tacitly admitted that the doctrine of mens rea could not be safely applied to the insane. A criminal lunatic might be as morally innocent as a man who had done harm by accident or in self-defense, but the danger of *treating* him as innocent was too great. The solution was to pay lip-service to his innocence but use the law to make sure he remained in custody. (ibid., 81)

Life imprisonment was a much stiffer sentence than short-term incarceration, but because it was still lighter than the death penalty, which was the usual punishment for homicide, some officials worried that murderers would simply feign madness in order to escape execution. This was by no means an ill-founded concern, because it appeared that a majority of "insane" killers regained their sanity very shortly after their arrest, thus making their illness highly suspect. The following homicide, tried in 1760, is a case in point:

In 1760, the Board of Punishments, in conjunction with the Censorate and the Court of Revision, deliberated a case submitted to them by the governor of Jiangxi. According to the governor's report, Wu Yuanchang Zi, a resident of Yongfeng district, fatally wounded a woman by the name of Yang. The officials established the fact that Wu lost his father when he was a young child. His mother, woman Tao, subsequently re-married to a man named Xu Fuliu. Xu's first wife had a son, Xu Zusheng, who was married to the victim. The Xu family seemed to get along very well with Wu. Wu and Xu Zusheng, for example, enjoyed an amicable relationship, and the step-father liked Wu enough to arrange a marriage for him, to the daughter of a man named Lo Yulong.

During the summer of 1759, Wu suddenly became mad. His grandmother, woman Chen, thought that marriage would be the ideal treatment for his illness. She therefore approached Xu Fuliu and asked him to make the necessary arrangements with Lo. Lo, however, refused to give his consent, citing as excuse both his daughter's young age and Wu's illness. Subse-quently, Wu recovered from his illness, and soon afterwards expressed his intention to sell part of his patrimony in order to get married. He went over to Xu Fuliu's house to fetch his mother so that she could take part in the negotiations with his uncle, Wu Cuilu, over the sale of his share of the family land-holding. His uncle, however, would have nothing to do with Yuanchang Zi's proposal, claiming that he was still not well enough to undertake such a venture. The matter being thus settled, Tao returned to her husband's home. The same day, Wu Yuanchang Zi showed up at the Xu household, to ask his mother for money. Tao took out two hundred cash to give him, but she was intercepted by her stepdaughter-in-law, woman Yang. Tao subsequently gave Wu only one hundred cash; the other hundred she gave Yang to put away for her. Wu tried to snatch the money from Yang, but the woman would not let go. He then took hold of a vegetable knife that was lying on a nearby table and stabbed Yang with it. Yang col-lapsed onto the floor and died. Wu was arrested and confessed readily to his crime.

As far as the governor was concerned, the key point in the case was whether Wu was insane at the time of the murder. The governor's impression of Wu was that he only *appeared* to be mad, while in fact he was quite sane. His testimony, for example, was clear and coherent, unlike that of others who had completely lost their senses. Ultimately, the governor concluded that he could not try the case as homicide committed because of insanity. But was it premeditated murder? The struggle between Wu and Yang over the money, in the governor's opinion, had all the elements of an affray. Wu, during the struggle, and without forethought, grabbed a knife and stabbed the woman with it. It was not premeditated murder (*mousha*), but homicide committed during an affray (*dousha*). The governor therefore recommended the statutory sentence for the offense, strangulation after the assizes. The officials in Beijing upheld the governor's recommendation. They pointed out, however, that because the governor had already determined that Wu did not commit homicide because of insanity, his relatives, as well as the village constable, should not be held responsible for his crime. This decision was ultimately approved by the Qianlong emperor (*Cheng'an xinpian* 1763, 9:12a–13a).

As they wrestled with the possibility of criminal abuse of the system, Qing judicial officials once again turned to the mandatory registration-and-confinement laws. They recognized that statutory procedures relating to registration provided them with a ready-made (and perhaps fail-safe) means to ascertain the veracity of a criminal's insanity claim. Thus, in 1802, the Board of Punishments notified provincial officials that the only indisputable proof of insanity was prior registration with the authorities. In cases where such proof was available, the murderers would be tried under the 1762 substatute and sentenced to life imprisonment.

Qing jurists did not dismiss outright the claims of those who had not been previously registered as officially insane. They appeared to accept the possibility that a person might suddenly become murderously crazed. They were also inclined to accept that lucidity might not be a good test for sanity because of the episodic nature of madness, a characteristic that was well documented in medical texts. However, they insisted that these claims had to be corroborated by testimony provided by the victim's family. In the end, therefore, jurists allowed their skepticism to triumph, for they offered this category of murderers only the relatively lighter death sentence of strangulation after the assizes! On the other hand, the sentence for a murderer who could not obtain corroborating testimony from the victim's family was even worse: decapitation after the assizes (*Xing'an huilan* 1968, 2114, 2117). The 1802 directive at first seemed satisfactory, for it met three needs. First, it gave the mandatory registration-and-confinement scheme a much-needed reinforcement. Second, it allayed the fears of those who were concerned that the official lenient policy toward insane killers might encourage "hardened criminals" to exploit the system, because they too would now have to face the possibility of execution. Third, by providing the arrested murderers a chance to substantiate their claims of insanity, and by stipulating for them the relatively lighter sentence of strangulation after the assizes, the directive satisfied, albeit tenuously, the time-honored principle of showing clemency toward the inadvertent offender. In addition, because the death sentence was to be reviewed during the Autumn Assizes, there was always the possibility that the judges would defer the execution. Because of all these positive aspects, the directive was formally incorporated into the Qing Code as a substatute in 1806 (ibid., 1968, 2114, 2117). The following is an example of the 1806 law in action:

In 1811, the Shandong department of the Board of Punishments reviewed a homicide case involving a man by the name of Hou Fa. Hou's younger brother, Hou Cunyi, had died some years earlier without having fathered a son. His widow, woman Dou, adopted a distant member of the family, Hou San, to be her son and heir. One day, Hou Fa came across an anonymous note which insinuated that Dou was having an affair with her adopted son. Hou Fa shredded the note on the spot and then went home to confront his sister-in-law about the alleged affair. She denied the illicit liaison, but Hou Fa did not believe her. He brooded over the accusation so much that he became insane, and was given to unpredictable outbursts of laughter and tears. One day, during one such fit of madness, he took a vegetable knife with him to a neighbor's house, killed the neighbor, woman Zheng, and seriously wounded her daughter, who died more than ten days later (a circumstance that, according to Qing law, dissociated her death from the original infliction of injury). When Hou Fa was apprehended, he still had not regained his senses. Only after he was imprisoned, and a physician was brought in to treat him, did he finally recover enough to give a coherent confession. The district magistrate was able to obtain statements from the victim's family as well as from his neighbors, who all vouched that Hou Fa was genuinely insane. The magistrate's tentative sentence was strangulation after the assizes, as stipulated by the substatute of 1806. The Board of Punishments concurred (*Shuotie leipian* 1835, 22:29a–29b; see also *Xing'an huilan* 1968, 2112–13).

Within a few decades, however, Qing officials began to have qualms about the 1806 law. Specifically, they were uneasy about the insistence that only prior registration could be considered indisputable proof of insanity. It had become apparent by the mid-nineteenth century that the mandatory registration-and-confinement laws were heeded by only a small percentage of affected households. Most of the apprehended "insane" murderers were unregistered and had to rely on their victim's family to support their insanity claims—a most unlikely eventuality. Moreover, even if they succeeded in securing such support, the government would still not regard the testimony as sufficient proof of insanity; this was why the 1806 substatute (and its predecessor, the 1802 directive) stipulated the sentence of strangulation after the assizes. They would still face the possibility of execution. For these convicts and their families the distinction between strangulation and decapitation was only a formal one, for it was only of small comfort for them to know that they could remain filial to their parents by keeping their bodies intact.

Since it was not the intention of the government to punish genuinely insane criminals, let alone execute them, in 1852 a new law was enacted to supersede the 1806 substatute. The new law abandoned the prior-registration condition, and substituted instead incoherency as the standard test of insanity. It stipulated that murderers who remained incoherent after their arrest, and therefore could not testify in their own behalf, would not be tried. Instead, they would be remanded to prison for a period of two to three years. If they regained their sanity during this waiting period, they would be brought to trial and, if convicted, given the statutory sentence of strangulation after the assizes. Murderers who regained their sanity shortly after their arrest would be brought to trial immediately and given the sentence of strangulation after the assizes as well. These sentences, however, were only pro forma, because the law stated that they would be ruled "deferred" at the assizes. In other words, insane killers who "recovered" within the three-year waiting period were in actuality condemned to life imprisonment. Those who failed to recover within the stipulated period would not ever have to face trial; however, neither would they ever be released from prison (Nakamura 1973, 193).

The substatute of 1852 effectively killed five birds with one stone. First, by keeping the statutory death sentence for convicted insane murderers, it satisfied the demands of those who wanted a-life-for-a-life restitution for the homicide. Second, it nevertheless eliminated the possibility of executing genuinely insane criminals. Third, it guaranteed at least long-term imprisonment for successful fakers. Fourth, it ensured that only those who were competent to stand trial were actually brought to trial, thus realizing the principle that punishment should be inflicted only on those who could comprehend its significance. Fifth—and this was an important consideration—by stipulating virtual life imprisonment for the insane murderer, this law ensured that the criminally insane would be segregated from the rest of society, thus neutralizing their threat to public safety. The jurists had accomplished a remarkable balancing act. This substatute is even more remarkable when we take into account the fact that the catastrophic Taiping Rebellion by this time was into its second year and showing no signs of abating. That Board of Punishments officials would still be agonizing over the possibility of putting to death a genuinely insane killer shows that they were able to maintain their sense of justice even at a time of tremendous dynastic stress. To their credit, too, even as the rebellion waged on, there were no subsequent attempts to pursue a harder line with respect to single homicides committed by the insane. (In contrast, as was shown earlier in this chapter, treason and parricide incurred more vengeful responses during dynastic crises because their subversive nature rendered them more dangerous when the state was being challenged.)

Enactment of a "perfect" law did not spell the end to uncertainties. The key question remained the same: Was the murderer insane at the time of the killing? As was pointed out in Chapter Two, much depended on rather idiosyncratic interpretations by the judicial officials involved. Moreover, the specter of the insanity plea being exploited by hard-nosed criminals continued to loom large over the trials. In 1853, for example, the Zhili department of the Board of Punishments reviewed the transcripts of a homicide trial:

Chen Yongxiang had a long history of episodic madness. He shared living quarters in a Guanyin temple with a Daoist priest by the name of Zhao Fuyi. One evening in 1853, Chen returned to the temple just when Zhao was getting ready to go to bed. Zhao immediately began to berate Chen for having stayed out too late, but Chen took his scolding in stride. Zhao continued his tirade, telling Chen that because there was no one to watch the place during the cold weather, he should move out the next day and seek lodging elsewhere. At that point, Chen began to argue with Zhao and a bitter quarrel ensued. Zhao even threw a piece of brick at Chen. The aggravation proved to be too much for Chen, and his madness returned. He, too, picked up a piece of brick and used it to hit Zhao several times. He also struck Zhao on the head with the bracket of an iron bucket, killing him instantly.

The next day, with the murder weapon in his hand, Chen took to the streets and danced up and down in a wild manner. It so happened that one of Zhao's acquaintances, a man by the name of Zhang Fengnian, was in the neighborhood. When he saw Chen acting so strangely, he decided to see Zhao about it. It was thus that he found Zhao's body, lying naked alongside the *kang* (heatable brick bed). It also appeared that Zhao's bedding, as well as all his clothes, had been taken from the room. Suspecting that Chen was somehow implicated, Zhang nabbed the crazed man and took him to the magistrate's yamen. During subsequent interrogations at both the district and provincial levels, Chen was able to testify in a coherent manner. Convinced that Chen was insane at the time of the murder, the governor-general of Zhili recommended the sentence of strangulation after the assizes, as was prescribed by the substatute of 1852.

The officials at the Board of Punishments, however, seemed predisposed to be suspicious of Chen's claim of insanity. In their own summation of the case, they noted several questionable aspects. First, Chen's illness had not been registered with the district magistrate. Second, the incident took place in the middle of the night, thus there were no eyewitnesses who could substantiate that Chen was insane at the time of the killing. Third, it was inconceivable that Chen could land so many blows on Zhao without the latter's hitting him once in return. The fact that Chen did not have any wounds on his body should, therefore, cast doubt on his assertion that the two had been involved in an affray. And fourth, since Chen remained in the vicinity of the temple during the night and the next day as well, it was impossible for a burglar to sneak into the temple to steal Zhao's bedding and clothing.

The board officials concluded that Chen killed Zhao while the latter was sound asleep in order to steal his personal effects. Afterwards, he feigned madness in order to escape more severe punishment. Having reached such a conclusion, the board reprimanded the provincial officials for having failed to investigate every aspect of the case, thereby allowing themselves to be duped by the criminal. A retrial was ordered (*Xing'an huilan xupian* 1970, 3024–26).

Sometimes, their suspicions notwithstanding, Board of Punishments officials elected to err on the side of leniency. For example, in 1860, the governor of Anhui submitted a memorial regarding a case of homicide committed by Su Zhaoqing, a former sergeant in the Anhui army. According to the governor, Su subsequently recovered fully from his illness and was even able to fight valiantly in a number of battles. It was Su's military record that moved the governor to recommend to the Board of Punishments that Su be given a light sentence. Board officials, however, were skeptical about the facts of the case:

> We have examined carefully the particulars of this case. Su Zhaoqing, because of insanity, fatally wounded Wu Yinglin. He was given medical care and was thus able to regain complete control of his faculties. His recovery was so complete that he subsequently compiled a record of valor in the battlefield. In our opinion it is highly probable that he feigned madness in order to hide the fact that the murder was premeditated.
>
> Moreover, Su Zhaoqing committed his crime during the summer of 1858; yet, although his victim was an official, there had been no attempt at the time to report the case to the Board of Punishments. What was the reason for this concealment? The fact of his subsequent stint in the army was also not reported. Now, more than two years after the homicide, the governor is recommending special treatment for him, citing as reason his army record. It is obvious to us that the governor delayed reporting the crime in order to build up a strong case in Su's favor (*Xing'an huilan xupian* 1970, 5008).

Having thus registered their suspicions about the governor's actions, the board rejected his plea on behalf of Su Zhaoqing. Instead, the board issued the order that Su be remanded to prison for at least five years, at the end of which time he would be examined to determine if he had fully recovered from his illness and statutory procedures necessary to process his possible release could then be initiated. It is noteworthy that the board did not reject outright the claim of insanity; had they done so Su would have been sentenced to death. Even more intriguing is the fact that the board did not apply the 1852 substatute to the case. The five-year stipulation could have been inspired by the 1808 substatute that governed amnesties (see Chapter Five), but surely board officials could not have intended to treat Su Zhaoqing as one who had received an imperial pardon! Unfortunately, the memorandum that summed up this case did not offer any explanations.

Another question begs to be answered: If officials were so concerned about fraudulent claims of insanity, why did they not stipulate that medical experts be included in the evaluative process? By the Qing period there was a sophisticated system of medical ideas concerning madness, and a number of influential Qing physicians had in fact made their own distinctive contributions to the collective knowledge on the subject. One possible explanation is that during this period physicians were held in such low esteem that it did not occur to Board of Punishments officials to solicit their professional opinion. For example, Sybille van der Sprenkel is of the opinion that "Chinese medical and scientific knowledge [were not] advanced enough to be of assistance in assessing evidence (or, if the level of knowledge reached was enough, it was not harnessed. . . .)" (1977, 74). In any case, in the absence of objective assessment of an accused's claim of insanity judicial officials had no recourse but to rely on their own experience and instincts. Their suspicions were most acute when possible motives could be discerned, as the following case reviewed in 1854 by the Zhili department of the Board of Punishments shows:

Yu Sheng first became afflicted with episodic madness when he was about fourteen; however, his condition was never reported to the proper authorities. One day in 1854, while his mother was away visiting her relatives, Yu decided to go out to the fields to dig up some vegetables. Passing an ironware dealer, he suddenly realized that the knife he was carrying was not suitable for his task, so he bought a different sort of implement—in fact, a short-handled sword—from the dealer.

It was a stiflingly hot day. The heat was so oppressive that Yu suddenly lost control of his senses. Running to the fields, he attacked the owner of one of the vegetable plots, slashing the hapless man with his newly bought sword. His mad rampage did not end until he had lopped off his victim's head and disemboweled him as well. Yu then went off to the bank of a nearby river, lay down on the ground, and fell asleep. When he woke up during the early part of the evening, he felt that his head had cleared somewhat and so he returned to the village. He was subsequently arrested and brought to trial. The governor-general of Zhili found him to have been insane at the time of the murder and recommended the sentence of strangulation after the assizes, as was prescribed by the substatute of 1852. The officials at the Zhili department of the Board of Punishments, however, felt that the governor-general had been too ready to accept the words of a murderer. But their own logic was a bit twisted. The criminal had a long history of episodic madness, they noted, so it was only a matter of time before he got himself into trouble. Even though his condition was not reported to the proper authorities, and he was therefore not held in confinement, someone should have been keeping an eye on him. In any case, they insisted, it seemed inconceivable that he had not premeditated the murder. The criminal claimed that he left his house with knife in hand because he wanted to go to the fields to dig up some vegetables, and that he bought the murder weapon from the dealer only because he realized that his knife was not suitable. He was obviously bending the facts to save himself!

The board officials continued: Even if one accepted that Yu had a long history of madness, how could one explain the fact that he was in perfect control of himself when he purchased the sword, only to turn into a raving, homicidal maniac almost immediately afterwards? His claim of insanity simply was not convincing. In fact, the extraordinary brutality of his crime suggested the possibility that the murder was motivated by a deep-seated grudge or hatred, and that he feigned madness after the fact solely to escape more severe punishment. The provincial officials had not investigated the case carefully enough and had allowed themselves to be fooled by the cunning words of the criminal. They should reopen their investigation of the case (*Xing'an huilan xupian* 1970, 3027–29).

In this case the criminal's murderous abandonment was interpreted as having been motivated by his hatred for the victim. Lest one jumps to the immediate conclusion that Qing jurists did not accept the "irresistible impulse" test of insanity, consider the following case, reported to the Board of Punishments in 1867 by the military governor of Rehe:

Han Ming, the criminal in the case, had once been in the

employ of his murder victim, woman Zhao. Although Han had a history of episodic madness, he had not previously caused any trouble because of his illness. He was a spendthrift, and when he was out of money he often turned to Zhao for a loan, pledging his clothes as security. Whenever Zhao rejected his loan request—and this happened quite often—he would argue with her so fiercely that his boss, Liu Yingxiao, often had to order him to quiet down. Subsequently, Han was without explanation dismissed by Liu. Convinced that Zhao was responsible for his unemployment, Han paid her a visit, hoping that a sincere apology would placate her and, perhaps, give him his job back. Zhao, however, refused to have anything to do with him. Feeling deeply humiliated, Han suddenly suffered a relapse of his illness. He grabbed a nearby knife, stabbed Zhao once, and then turned the knife on himself. He collapsed onto the floor, his eyes staring blankly ahead. Zhao staggered outside the house and into the arms of her stunned husband. She managed to mention Han's name before she expired. Han was arrested and brought to trial. The military governor of Rehe applied the substatute of 1852 to the case and recommended the sentence of strangulation after the assizes.

When the officials at the Board of Punishments examined the particulars of the case, they found that several aspects required more thorough examination. For example, regarding the purpose of Han's visit with Zhao, the officials had only the criminal's statement to rely on. Since Liu was not present at the time, and Zhao did not manage to tell her husband the reason for Han's visit, there was no one to confirm Han's testimony. What could not be denied was the fact that the relationship between Han and Zhao had not been good, and Han himself admitted his suspicions about Zhao's complicity in his dismissal. Clearly, the board officials noted, this suggested that he harbored a grudge against the woman. Moreover, Han had already confessed that he became insanely angry after Zhao spurned his fence-mending attempt; this pointed to the possibility that he killed her in order to avenge his humiliation. More importantly, in the officials' opinion, Han stabbed his victim only once. This meant that he had taken such deadly aim and was so sure that he had killed the woman that he did not bother to stab her again. His self-inflicted wounds and subsequent collapse were all part of a masquerade designed to dupe the investigating officials. Indeed, emphasized the board officials, all the information contained in the military governor's report pointed to the fact that Han Ming was not at all befuddled. The officials were also very critical of the slipshod quality of the military governor's report. They pointed out that it did not contain bonded statements from neighbors and the local constable, nor did it state whether Liu's shop was situated in an area where there were neighbors. Also, the report did not describe the condition of the corpse or the location of the murder weapon, thus it was not clear whether the knife was found near the *kang* upon which woman Zhao died, or in Han's hand. The nature of the criminal's self-inflicted wounds, too, was unclear. The board ordered the military governor to reopen the investigation in order to obtain detailed statements from all the material witnesses, so that the case could be adjudicated properly (*Xing'an huilan xupian* (1970, 3003–3005).

Multiple Homicide

The decision to punish or not to punish hung on a delicate balance, one that could easily be tipped. Although jurists managed to convince themselves that a-life-for-a-life retribution was unjust to insane criminals found guilty of single homicide, it was by no means automatic that they would extend such magnanimity to those guilty of multiple homicide. After all, in Qing law, multiple homicide was a very grievous offense, one that warranted the ultimate penalty, *lingchi*. The earliest documented evidence of movement toward a harsher position was a memorial submitted in 1766 by Shi Lijia, the judicial commissioner of Sichuan. He had just presided over the trial of a madman who was accused of murdering four people, and he had become very disturbed by the case, particularly because the victims were all from the same family. He would have liked to sentence the convicted killer to death, but he was prohibited by law from doing so. The maximum sentence he could impose on the insane murderer was, as stipulated by the homicide substatute of 1762, life imprisonment and a fine of 12.42 taels of silver. No distinction was made between single and multiple homicide in the substatute. After the conclusion of the case, Shi resolved to prevent insane criminals found guilty of committing multiple homicide from receiving such lenient treatment in the future. He thus submitted a memorial to the Qianlong emperor.

In his memorial, Shi conceded the rightness of sparing the life of an insane person found guilty of killing one, or even two people. He argued, however, that this leniency should not be extended to those who killed three or more people, especially when the victims were members of the same family. He insisted that consideration should be given to the fact that so many innocent lives were needlessly and tragically ended. In some instances, he noted, when the victims included all the male members of a family, an entire descent line could be terminated. A tragedy of such magnitude could not be rectified by life imprisonment and a fine. He therefore proposed that in the future, multiple homicide (involving three or more victims) committed by the insane should be made punishable by death.

The Board of Punishments, however, disagreed with the judicial commissioner of Sichuan. Board officials in fact criticized Shi for his failure to understand that the key issue was criminal responsibility of the insane, not the number of slain victims nor compassion for the victims and their families. The board insisted, "We must pardon inadvertent transgressions however grave they might be. It is for this reason that although the board has always felt sorry for the victims of multiple homicide committed by insane persons, we have so far refrained from punishing their killers more severely than those who had taken only one life." Putting to death insane murderers guilty of multiple homicide would only be an act of retribution, in which case justice would not be served. Moreover, the board asked, if the judicial commissioner was so concerned about the victims, how would he justify his exclusion of homicides with fewer than three victims from his proposal for heavier penalties? A more appropriate response to the problem of insanity-related homicide, the board suggested, would be to intensify efforts to seek out and identify insane persons who were still at large, so they could be placed under surveillance and control (*Dingli huipian* 1762–1883, 13:73a–73b). The mandatory registration-and-confinement substatute of 1766 was, in fact, an unanticipated outcome of the efforts of the Sichuan judicial commissioner to seek redress for victims of multiple homicide.

Ten years later, in 1776, one of the presidents of the Censorate, Cui Yinggai, initiated another round of discussion about the matter. Cui was even more unsympathetic toward insane murderers than was Shi Lijia, for he proposed that those found guilty of double homicide be sentenced to strangulation after the assizes, with the proviso that they be found "deserving of punishment" (*qingshi*) at the assizes. In other words, he wanted to ensure that their sentences would not be reprieved at the Autumn Assizes.

Cui's arguments were essentially the same as those of Shi—sympathy for the victims and so forth—but, perhaps mindful of the board's response to Shi's proposal in 1766, he specifically addressed only the crime of double homicide, thus skirting adroitly the numbers game. Cui's status within the central government no doubt also lent his proposal more weight than a similar recommendation from a provincial official. In any case, the Board of Punishments, in a drastic departure from the position taken ten years earlier, agreed that consideration should be given to the victims. Such being the case, it was truly a miscarriage of justice to allow their killers to live on in prison without ever having to endure the ordeals of receiving the death sentence and the lengthy (and tortuous) process of judicial review. The board had not abandoned the time-honored notion that insane criminals were inadvertent offenders, but they now reasoned that although these murderers were not aware of their actions, the fact remained that they did kill people with their own hands, thus making them liable for punishment. However, in spite of their new hard line, the board could not be prevailed upon to accept Cui's recommendation that the proviso "deserving of punishment" be added to the death sentence. The board pointed out that only the officials presiding at the assizes had the authority to decide the ultimate fate of a criminal (ibid., 14:40a–41b).

What accounted for the change in attitude? A change in personnel in the Board of Punishments might be a partial reason, but in the absence of information about the names and backgrounds of board officials who participated in the deliberations, this will have to remain a matter of speculation. Another contributing cause might be the 1774 Wang Lun uprising in Shandong, the first major sectarian challenge to the Qianlong reign, which had fractured the Qing's peaceful and harmonious self-image. It is possible that the violence attending the uprising moved judicial officials to adopt a harder line toward any sort of mass murder.

The position adopted by the Board of Punishments in 1776 marked a significant turning point in the evolution of Qing laws dealing with insane killers. Although officials still assumed that insane persons were not conscious of their actions, they had managed to overcome their earlier reluctance to sentence insane murderers to death. This was accomplished with the rationalization that they did kill people with their own hands. This new attitude not only affected multiple homicide, but had ramifications on single homicide as well. As was pointed out in the preceding section, single homicide committed by the insane was made a capital offense in 1802.

The new judicial position was translated into a substatute the same year. Like so many other laws relating to criminal insanity, it created more problems than the lawmakers had ever anticipated. It appeared that some officials found themselves in a judicial quandary. They were uncertain whether the substatute of 1776 applied only to double homicide or to multiple homicide in general. And because the substatute did not have any specific stipulation about cases involving victims who were all members of the same family, some officials were also uncertain whether such cases should be evaluated as more grievous than "ordinary" multiple homicide. The issue finally came to a head in 1824, when the governor-general of Zhili sought advice from the Board of Punishments regarding a case over which he was presiding. In this particular case, the insane murderer had hacked to death four members of a family. "How should I handle this case?" the governor-general asked.

In response to his query, the officials at the Board of Punishments reviewed their records and found only one case which could serve as a precedent of sorts. In this earlier case, concluded in 1809, an insane man who killed three distant relatives was given the sentence of immediate decapitation and was subsequently executed. Commenting on the 1809 case, the board officials noted that the sentence was excessively harsh. They regretted the fact that three innocent persons were killed, but at the same time they felt that the murderer's affliction should not have been overlooked or discounted. Therefore, the answer to the governor-general's question was that it would be inappropriate to apply the substatutes governing multiple homicide committed by sane murderers to cases involving the insane, because the statutory punishments were too severe (decapitation for killing three or more unrelated people, and *lingchi* for premeditated murder of three or more people from the same family).

The board officials concluded that a more comprehensive substatute for multiple homicide was called for, in order to standardize procedures for the treatment of insane murderers. They recommended the following additions to the 1776 substatute:

(1) The punishment for killing three or more persons not of the same family, or two persons of the same family, should be strangulation after the assizes, with the proviso that the criminal be found "deserving of punishment" at the assizes.

(2) The punishment for killing three or more persons of the same family should be decapitation after the assizes, with the proviso that the criminal be found "deserving of punishment" at the assizes.

(3) Criminals who were found to have feigned madness should be tried according to the regular statute or substatute appropriate to the circumstances.

These recommendations were subsequently incorporated

into the 1824 Qing Code as amendments to the 1776 sub-statute (*Xing'an huilan* 1968, 2125–26; Xue 1970, 862–63).

The evolution of homicide laws pertaining to the insane presents us with an excellent illustration of the Qing legislative process. Thomas Metzger has noted that lawmaking was a continuous and basic process of the Qing state: bureaucrats were constantly and flexibly making adjustments in response to tendencies toward deviancy (1973, 22). The experience presented above shows also that bureaucrats were engaged in a seemingly ceaseless effort to rectify what they perceived to be imperfections in laws, not only to deter tendencies toward deviancy but also to serve justice well. In the case of single homicides, officials translated justice to mean remaining true to the spirit of the ancient doctrine of mens rea, which established the tradition of clemency for inadvertent offenders. In the case of multiple homicides, justice meant also considering the victims whose lives had been tragically ended (a Qing version of the concept of "violation of civil rights" that is sometimes applied in the United States to indict individuals who have caused the death of others). In both cases, the notion of diminished responsibility was found to be acceptable and fair.

Amnesty and Criminal Insanity

The assize system adopted by the Qing meant that criminals awaiting final adjudication had to spend a long time in prison. At the beginning the Manchus continued the Ming practice of having Hot Weather Assizes and Autumn Assizes, but the former had a sporadic history of enforcement and appears to have been abandoned in the nineteenth century. The Autumn Assizes handled cases that called for "execution after the assizes," and were spectacular and elaborate affairs. According to Bodde and Morris:

> The Autumn Assizes were scheduled for a day within the first ten days of the eighth lunar month (sometime during September in Western reckoning, by which time, according to the Chinese calendar, autumn was already half over). Their locale was not far south of the [Tiananmen] or Gate of Heavenly Peace, along the west side of the broad . . . Esplanade of a

Thousand Paces which leads southward from the Tiananmen Square toward the main south gate of Peking.

Although the walls flanking the east and west sides of the Esplanade were each lined on their inner face by a row of small cell-like rooms, it would seem from the wording of the sources that the assizes were not held in these rooms at all (which would have been too small), but in the open air in front of them. There, on the appointed day, several tens of tables, topped by red cloth coverings, were set forth for the participating jurists, who included prominent officials from the Nine Chief Ministries . . . as well as other dignitaries such as the tutors of the imperial heir apparent.

This mixed body examined the "after the assizes" cases and confirmed or altered their provisional classifications. From the *Daqing huidian* (53/2a) we learn that the various stages of the proceedings were reported in a loud voice and "listened to by the multitude of the humble"—statements indicating that these highest judicial proceedings, like those in the lowest district court, were open to the public. . . .

Following the conclusion of the Autumn . . . Assizes, the results of the classifications then arrived at were submitted to the emperor so that he might examine them prior to a final climactic ceremony at which he confirmed the disposition of the various categories. For the Autumn Assizes this ceremony took place some sixty days before the winter solstice or around October 21. . . . At dawn [on the scheduled day], high officials, including presidents or vice-presidents of the nine ministries mentioned earlier, representatives of the Grand Secretariat (a kind of inner cabinet), and others, assembled in the Hall of Earnest Diligence . . . located in the northern part of the Forbidden City. To mark the solemnity of the occasion, all wore funeral garb of plain undecorated white, the Chinese color for mourning. Our sources describe in great detail each move that followed. We can summarize by saying that the sub-chancellor, kneeling, placed the lists of the condemned on a table in front of the dais on which the emperor was sitting. Apparently the lists included the names of all those placed in the three categories leading to reduced punishment, as well as the fourth category of "circumstances deserving of capital punishment." It was only for the latter, however, that the ceremony was of crucial importance.

Having received the lists, the emperor inspected them and indicated approval either by marking them himself with his vermillion brush or having a grand secretary do this on his behalf. In particular, with regard to the list of persons in the category of "circumstances deserving of punishment," he checked off . . . the names of those actually destined to die. . . . What happened to those whose names were not checked off? They were kept in prison to re-experience the ordeal a year later. Those guilty of family offenses, if they twice succeeded in escaping the vermillion brush, then had their classification changed to "deferred execution," and their death penalty was reduced to a lower punishment. If, however, the convicted belonged to the sub-categories of either officials or ordinary persons, they then had to escape the vermillion brush no less than ten times before achieving the status of "deferred execution." By the law of averages, obviously few persons could thus escape the brush ten times running unless, as seems likely, the names of some were in fact consistently arranged in such a manner as to insure that they would not be checked. (1973, 136–41)

This elaborate system evolved out of the concept of cosmic harmony that was developed centuries earlier during the Han dynasty (see Chapter One). To ensure such harmony, violations such as miscarriage of justice must be avoided, otherwise catastrophes might result. A practical result of this system, however, was that, as Bodde and Morris concluded, "although imprisonment was not recognized as a formal punishment in China, a great many people must nonetheless have spent a great deal of time in prison" (1973, 142). Insane criminals added to the prison population problem because by design they were in effect condemned to either life or long-term imprisonment.

Brian E. McKnight offers a provocative hypothesis regarding the genesis and evolution of the use of amnesty in imperial China. He accepts the traditional explanations for the uses of amnesty, such as show of imperial benevolence and rectification of cosmic imbalances; however, he suggests that the most compelling reason for the introduction and continuation of the amnesty system was to relieve prisons of the pressure of overpopulation (1981, chap. 6). The longstanding problem of overcrowded conditions was at times regarded by officials as a poor reason for the issuance of amnesties and pardons. Liu Song, a judicial official during the Jin dynasty (A.D. 280–420), wrote:

> In antiquity punishments were used to eliminate punishments; now the situation is the opposite. All the serious criminals who escape, if their hair has grown back out to be more than three inches long, suddenly [on being recaptured] are again shaved bald—this is using punishment to give birth to punishment. [Their sentences] are increased by a year. This is using penal servitude to give birth to penal servitude. Those who escape are a multitude; prisoners still held have accumulated in great numbers. Those who discuss it say, "As for those in custody, there is no way but for us to amnesty them." Repeatedly [their counsel] is followed and men are pardoned. . . . [After the decline of the Zhou] there were many troubles and for this reason [criminals] were pardoned and released. This was practiced provisionally and was certainly not a way of being kind to criminals! Arriving at the present it is constantly considered that crimes are piled up and cases are numerous. Amnesties are issued to disperse them. Therefore amnesties are excessively numerous and yet the jails are stuffed full. If this is not soon stopped it will be beyond help. (McKnight 1981, 117–18)

In spite of objections by officials such as Liu Song, this practice was continued into Qing times.

Life imprisonment was instituted for insane murderers in 1762, and for several decades they were denied the benefit of amnesties and pardons. No doubt a key factor in this was the concern of the government for public safety. It appeared that some officials felt that such a categorical exclusion was unfair; one of them, the governor of Shandong, took advantage of the general amnesty issued in 1796 by the new emperor, Jiaqing, to recommend a change in policy. The governor wisely did not try to secure the release of all insane prisoners, probably because he thought that such a sweeping proposal might not stand a chance of being approved. Instead, he argued the case only for those who had already served ten or twenty years of their life terms, as well as those who were over seventy years old. After some deliberation, the Board of Punishments recommended that insane prisoners seventy or older could be released from prison, regardless of how long they had been incarcerated. A prisoner under the age of seventy, in order to be considered for release, must have served at least twenty years of the life sentence. The board's position was approved by the emperor, thus allowing for the first time a number of insane prisoners to benefit from an act of grace.

Four years later, in 1800, insane prisoners were included for the first time in a clear-the-prisons edict. When the Jiaqing emperor issued the order, he specifically included criminals who were serving life sentences. Because it had the amnesty of 1796 as a precedent, the Board of Punishments promptly ordered the release of insane prisoners who had been incarcerated for more than twenty years, subject to certification of recovery. The board also compiled a list of insane inmates who did not meet the twenty-year prerequisite, and presented the list to the emperor for his adjudication. After examining the list, the emperor ordered the release of all insane criminals who had been imprisoned for five years or more, on the condition that they had fully recovered from their illness (*Zengding tongxing tiaoli* 1883, 1:25a–27a). The edict of 1800 set the precedent for future amnesties and clear-the-prisons declarations. There evolved three prerequisites for eligibility: full recovery from the illness; incarceration of at least five years since that recovery; and specific inclusion of the individual prisoner in the imperial edict. In 1808, the Qing lawmakers formulated a new substatute that formalized the procedures described above (Xue 1970, 861). Insane criminals also became eligible for reduction of sentences. As in the case of a general amnesty or pardon, they first had to satisfy the requirement that they had been fully recovered for at least five years (*Xing'an huilan xupian* 1970, 3008–3009; 3010–11; 3034–35).

The amnesty substatute added new wrinkles to what might have been more or less routine transactions. For example, in 1823, the Board of Punishments recommended to the Daoguang emperor that the sentence of Wang Liang, who critically wounded another man, be reduced from the statutory strangulation after the assizes to banishment. The reason they cited was that although Wang's victim did die of his wound several days afterwards, Wang's offense was not as grievous as that involving instant death. Because Wang was deemed genuinely insane, the board also recommended that instead of actually being sent into exile, he should serve out his sentence in prison.

The emperor was curious to know how prisoners like Wang should be treated when an amnesty was declared. According to established procedures, he noted, insane criminals whose formal sentence was the death penalty could be considered for release from prison if they had spent at least five illness-free years in prison. What might the policy be regarding criminals whose formal sentence was banishment? He therefore ordered the Statutes Commission to study the question and render an opinion as quickly as possible. The commission replied that in 1806 Peng Xiaosan, a native of Shandong province, during a fit of madness inflicted injury on his wife, who died more than ten days later, after the usual "healing period" had expired. Under ordinary circumstances—that is, if Peng had not been insane—the customary punishment for such an offense would have been exile. However, because Peng was insane, the governor of Shandong saw fit to sentence him to life imprisonment instead. His judgment was upheld by the Board of Punishments. The commissioners saw an analogy with the case under consideration. They also noted that insane criminals who were formally sentenced to exile had always been sent to prison instead, to serve de facto life terms. As for Wang, because he suffered from episodic bouts of madness, it would be impossible to guarantee that he would not suffer a relapse and cause more trouble in the future. It would therefore be unwise to dispatch him to the site of his exile.

Addressing Daoguang's question, the commissioners held that it was difficult for them to determine precisely how long Wang should be imprisoned before he could become a beneficiary of amnesty or pardon decrees; this was because they did not have any substatutes or precedents to go by. However, they offered a possible solution: since there were well-defined amnesty procedures for insane inmates who were serving life terms, it might be advisable to sentence Wang to a formal life term, rather than remanding him to prison to serve out his sentence of exile. If this sentencing approach was adopted, the Board of Punishments in the future would for all practical purposes have to address itself only to insane prisoners serving life sentences, thereby simplifying the entire amnesty review process. Daoguang found this recommendation reasonable and signalled his approval (*Xing'an huilan* 1968, 2115–16).

Case records reveal that prisoners whose names were not included in the official lists compiled by the Board of Punishments for imperial commutation could still take advantage of recent decrees of amnesty or pardon by petitioning the Board of Punishments for special consideration. For example, in 1819, the Shangdong department of the Board of Punishments considered the following case:

Wei Kun, an inmate serving a life sentence, petitioned the government to release him from prison on the grounds that he had fully recovered from his illness and that the Jiaqing emperor had proclaimed an amnesty earlier in the year, on New Year's Day. The board officials reviewed, first of all, the circumstances of Wei's imprisonment. They learned that Wei had killed his wife during a fit of madness nine years before, in 1810. Because he did not regain his senses after his arrest, and was therefore unable to testify coherently, he was remanded to prison. Although he suffered a relapse during the first five years of his imprisonment, from 1815 until he submitted his petition in 1819 he had been free from all symptoms of his illness. The officials reviewed next all the substatutes and precedents that might have bearing on the case. One of them was the 1762 homicide substatute, which stipulated that an insane criminal sentenced to life imprisonment could not be freed, even if he or she had fully recovered. Another was the 1801 substatute regarding *liuyang chengsi* (remaining at home to care for parents or to perpetuate the ancestral sacrifices), which stipulated that, in order to be eligible for release, the inmate must be completely free of all symptoms of mental illness and that the local officials must present bonded statements affirming his recovery. (This substatute will be discussed in Chapter Five.) Yet another law that had bearing on the case was the amnesty substatute of 1808.

After much careful consideration, the Board of Punishments ruled that the homicide substatute of 1762 precluded any possibility of Wei Kun's having his life sentence commuted. Therefore, it was inappropriate to use the amnesty of 1819 as the basis for his petition. However, because he stated that his son had died, leaving him the sole surviving member of his family, he could request permission to regain his freedom on the basis of *chengsi* (to continue ancestral sacrifices). The board instructed the governor of Shandong to ask the prison authorities to determine if Wei had completely recovered and to certify their finding in the form of a bonded statement. After these steps had been taken, the governor should then submit a memorial to the emperor, along with the pertinent supporting documents, to secure his permission to release Wei from prison for the purpose of *chengsi* (*Shuotie leipian* 1836, 2:41a–42b).

In 1848, the Shandong department considered another petition. Zhu Shu, already serving time in prison, was originally sentenced to death by strangulation for the offense of homicide commited during a fit of madness, but his execution was deferred at the Autumn Assizes. Early in 1831, the Daoguang emperor proclaimed an amnesty, and Zhu was among a number of capital offenders whose names were sent up for consideration. At that time, the Board of Punishments ruled that Zhu be kept in prison for five more years, after which time, if it could be determined that he had fully recovered, the amnesty of 1831 could be retroactively applied to him, and his situation would be evaluated according to established procedures. Subsequently, during the five-year period, there was another effort to reevaluate criminals whose sentences had been deferred at the Autumn Assizes. At this juncture, as well as in 1836 (the end of the stipulated five-year period) it was determined that Zhu had not yet fully recovered, thus no positive action was taken in his behalf. However, the Board of Punishments did rule that his condition would be looked into periodically.

In 1848, the governor of Shandong reported to the board that Zhu had not suffered a relapse for more than five years. He noted that, in light of the history of his case, Zhu's death sentence should, at the very least, be reduced to exile. But since Zhu had been the subject of two reduction-of-sentence amnesties, it might be possible to reduce his sentence even further. It was to ponder this possibility that the Shandong department of the Board of Punishment met to consider this case.

During the process of review, the board officials discovered that at the 1831 amnesty the Board of Punishments acted to reduce the sentences of two inmates—Liu Hu and Cao Minming, who were serving time in prison for homicide committed during a fit of madness—from deferred strangulation to exile. Both Liu and Cao had spent more than five years in prison and had already recovered. One year later, in 1832, when the Daoguang emperor proclaimed another amnesty, their sentences of exile were further reduced to one hundred blows with heavy bamboo plus three years of penal servitude. Liu's case was disposed of in 1834 (meaning that he was released from prison?). In 1836 the emperor proclaimed yet another amnesty, thus Cao's sentence was further reduced to one hundred blows. His case was disposed of in 1837.

Regarding the case in question, the board officials were of the opinion that Zhu Shu's situation was similar to those of both Liu and Cao, so it was possible for him to benefit from the cumulative results of the series of amnesties proclaimed during the time he was imprisoned. The board calculated that in 1831 his original death sentence was reduced to one hundred blows plus exile to a location three thousand li away. In 1845 and 1846, two additional amnesties were proclaimed, effectively further reducing his sentence to one hundred blows plus payment of 12.42 taels of silver to his victim's family. The board decided that such should be his status in 1848 (*Xing'an huilan xupian* 1970, 3033–36).

Among all the criminal cases scrutinized for this study,

those dealing with petitions for pardons reveal the highest degree of tentativeness on the part of the judicial officials. One reason for this may be that unlike other more clear-cut cases which address specific offenses, the amnesty/pardon cases involve criminals imprisoned for a variety of reasons; this meant that the officials had to consider not only the specific amnesty/pardon decree that instigated the petition but also the nature of the original offense, as well as other pertinent factors. The following are two more examples:

In 1849 the Henan department of the Board of Punishments considered the case of Tang Baoshan, an inmate convicted eight years earlier of killing another man during a fit of madness. Tang was sentenced to death by strangulation but, by 1849, his execution had already been deferred seven times. The question the department was asked to consider was this: Since Tang's death sentence had already been deferred seven times, should his sentence be reduced? The board officials replied that Tang was not yet eligible to have his sentence adjusted. Criminals in his situation could have their sentences reevaluated only if an imperial edict of amnesty specifically included them among the beneficiaries of the act of grace. In the absence of such a decree, criminals like Tang needed to have their death sentences deferred *twenty* times before they could be eligible to benefit from reduction-of-sentence decrees. As for Tang, because his death sentence had been deferred only seven times, and because there had not been any edict that called for the adjustment of sentences of criminals of his kind, his situation should remain unchanged (*Xing'an huilan xupian* 1970, 3036–37).

In 1858 the Shandong department of the Board of Punishments considered the case of woman Li, a native of Shandong province, who was sentenced to immediate decapitation for cutting off her husband's penis, which resulted in his death. Because she was insane at the time of the incident, her sentence was reduced by the Xianfeng emperor to decapitation after the assizes. During the Autumn Assizes of 1854, Li was found to be "deserving of punishment," but because her name was not among those checked by the emperor, her execution was deferred. Later that same year, because of unrest in the province of Shandong, prisoners there, except those earmarked for execution, had their sentences formally reduced and were dispatched elsewhere. This was an emergency measure employed to clear the prisons of inmates. Li's death sentence was reduced to military exile, but because she was classified as an insane killer, the Board of Punishments ruled that she had to remain incarcerated until five years had elapsed since the last episode of her illness.

Now, in 1848, the governor of Shandong reported to the Board of Punishments that Li had not suffered a relapse during her five years in prison, therefore she should be ready to serve out her sentence of military exile. At the same time, however, the governor admitted to being confused about two separate provisions in the Qing Code and asked the board for advice. The code, he noted, allowed women sentenced to banishment to pay a monetary redemption in lieu of actually serving out the sentence; however, the code also stipulated that a woman guilty of killing her husband must remain in prison for life even if her death sentence had been deferred. Should Li be allowed to redeem her military exile sentence and be sent home, or should she be held in prison for life?

The board officials replied that, according to the bylaws established earlier in Zhili, in the event of a clear-the-prisons edict, all inmates, with the exception of those convicted of homicide committed during a fit of madness, and those thieves whose loot had not yet been fully recovered, would have their sentences reduced and summarily be dispatched. However, the insane killers referred to in the bylaws were actually those who had not yet fully recovered. These prisoners could not be allowed to leave because they might cause trouble once they were outside.

The officials noted that under normal circumstances, a woman guilty of killing her husband during a fit of madness could not be released from prison, even if she had fully recovered. (This subject will be discussed further in Chapter Five.) However, the clear-the-prisons decree issued for Shandong in 1854 was occasioned by the critical situation there. Because of widespread unrest in the province, there was fear that criminal elements in the provincial jails might take advantage of the situation to create trouble. At the same time, there was genuine concern that bandit troops might storm the local jails, resulting in massacres of hapless inmates. For these two reasons, it was deemed advisable to dispatch inmates elsewhere, away from Shandong. To accomplish this, the regular laws and precedents had been temporarily suspended. Because all categories of serious offenders were included in this clear-the-prisons decree, the board ruled at the time that it would be unfair to exclude Li from it, particularly since she had recovered. It was thus that the officials reduced her sentence to military exile in spite of the fact that a substatute in the Qing Code specifically prohibited women guilty of killing their husbands from being released from prison.

As to the specific query of the governor of Shandong, the board ruled that, since Li had already spent five years in prison, during which time she had not suffered a relapse of her illness, she should be allowed to serve out her exile sentence. Additionally, because the Qing Code allowed women to pay a monetary redemption in lieu of actual exile, woman Li should be permitted to do the same and be released to the protective custody of her family.

The board officials took one further step. They ruled that, since the Shandong governor had misunderstood the terms of the clear-the-prisons edict of 1854, it was possible that officials in other provinces that had experienced unrest might have committed the same mistake. They should be instructed to follow the Zhili bylaws, so that there would be uniform disposition of prisoners in all the affected provinces. However, provinces that were not affected by unrest should not apply the said bylaws. This decision was then sent out to the provinces by way of a general circular (*Xing'an huilan xupian* 1970, 3039–42).

The laws and procedures—and sometimes the circumstances themselves—were confusing enough, but when we add the ingredient of bureaucratic turf battle as well, we have a recipe for chaos. The following is a wondrously confusing example:

In 1870, the Fengtian department of the Board of Punishments considered the case of Zhang Zhiyou, who, because of insanity, killed two men. He regained his senses shortly after his arrest, testified, and was given the sentence of strangulation after the assizes. Subsequently, the prison where he was held was raided by a gang of bandits. Because he did not participate in the general rampage that ensued, Zhang's sentence was reduced to one hundred blows with heavy bamboo plus exile to a location three thousand li away. One of the vice presidents of the Manchurian Board of Punishments, without waiting for final approval by the Board of Punishments in Beijing, proceeded immediately to dispatch Zhang to his place of exile. (Note: Manchuria—made up of Heilongjiang, Kirin, and Fengtian—the original home of the Manchus, had its own centralized administration. This administration included, among its organs, a Board of Punishments for Manchuria which was separate from the Board of Punishments in Beijing. However, cases originating in Manchuria had to go to Beijing for final approval, as they did from the provinces of China proper [Bodde and Morris 1973, 121–23].)

When the officials in Beijing were able to review the case, however, they found fault with the actions taken by the Manchurian judicial official. They pointed out that Zhang was a bannerman and, as such, should have his original sentence reduced to canguing, rather than banishment. They also noted that Zhang had not yet served enough years in prison to make him eligible for release. Moreover, the Manchurian official had failed to obtain and forward to Beijing the requisite bonded statement from the prison officials before dispatching Zhang to his place of exile. This oversight was in violation of the stipulations of the relevant homicide law. The Board of Punishments in Beijing instructed their Manchurian counterpart to ascertain carefully the particulars of the case and to submit a detailed report of their investigation to Beijing. It was this report that the Fengtian department reviewed in 1870.

The vice president of the Manchurian Board of Punishments defended his decision to send Zhang to his place of exile without waiting for approval from the Beijing officials. He pointed out that in Zhang's original confession he stated only that he was from Beijing and had made no mention of the prince under whom he served or his own banner captain. In other words, he was befuddled as far as his banner identity was concerned. The vice president further noted that the penalty for such confusion, as stipulated by law, was banishment. The main reason for his decision to exile Zhang was that, in his opinion, Zhang's offense was too serious to be made punishable only by canguing. Thus, for the sake of making the punishment fit the crime, he had decided to apply the substatute "confusing one's banner captain" to the case and sentenced Zhang accordingly.

The vice president also reported that, after he received the reduction-of-sentence instructions from the Board of Punishments in Beijing, he did obtain bonded statements from prison officials who were familiar with Zhang's situation. They testified that he had not suffered a relapse of his illness since 1865, the year of his imprisonment. The vice president explained that he did not forward these statements to the board in Beijing because he was coping with the aftermath of the bandit raid on the prison, and also he did not have the benefit of precedents to guide his action.

The Fengtian department of the Board of Punishments responded as follows to the vice president's second report:

In homicide cases involving the insane, the relevant substatute stipulates that those who regained their senses and could testify in a coherent manner should be sentenced to [strangulation], and their cases reviewed at the Autumn Assizes. In the event that these offenders become eligible to have their sentences re duced, established procedures require that provincial officials calculate the number of years these criminals have already been imprisoned, up to the day of the receipt of the reduction decree. Under this reckoning, those who have already been incarcerated for five full years, and who have not suffered a relapse of their illness during this time, can have their sentences adjusted accordingly. However, the provincial officials must first submit bonded statements to the Board of Punishments along with their own reports before action on the case can be initiated. In this particular case, Zhang Ziyou, because of insanity, killed two persons. He was originally given the sentence of strangulation after the assizes, but because he did not participate in the unrest sparked by a bandit raid on the prison, his death sentence was subsequently reduced to banishment. In the opinion of the vice president of the Manchurian Board of Punishments, because Zhang killed two persons and wounded five others, it is inappropriate to reduce his sentence to canguing, for such punishment does not reflect the serious nature of the crime. A more appropriate sentence, in his opinion, is actual banishment. We concede that the vice president's point is well taken. The problem, however, is that the vice president cites, for the purpose of sentencing, the substatute "confusing one's banner captain." No such law exists in the Qing Code. Moreover, the criminal in question has not yet spent five full years in prison. Furthermore, the vice president has not obtained bonded statements concerning the criminal's state of health from the prison officials. [Note: The Manchurian official claimed that he had done so.] These statements should have been forwarded to the Board of Punishments in Beijing, which has the authority to decide the location of his place of exile. The vice president has acted contrary to the stipulations of existing laws.

The vice president should be instructed to follow established procedures. The criminal, Zhang Ziyou, should be remanded to prison until he has served fully five years of his term. When he has fulfilled this requirement, bonded statements concerning his state of health should be taken and forwarded to this board of review. (*Xing'an huilan xupian* 1970, 3019–22)

One cannot help but suspect that the issue in this case was not the fate of the criminal. It appears that he had the misfortune of being made a pawn in a turf struggle between the two boards of punishments.

Although the application of the amnesty/pardon substatute and procedures often produced confusion, the intent of the law and procedures themselves is clear. Insane convicts would have the same opportunity as other prisoners to benefit from the periodic issuance of acts of imperial grace, with the proviso that they had already served at least five years of their prison term and that they had not suffered a relapse during those five years. This additional stipulation was not a product of malicious intent but of genuine concern for the safety of the public. However, the effect of the minimum requirement of five years in prison meant that once the insane had been segregated from society, reintegration was more difficult than for other prisoners.

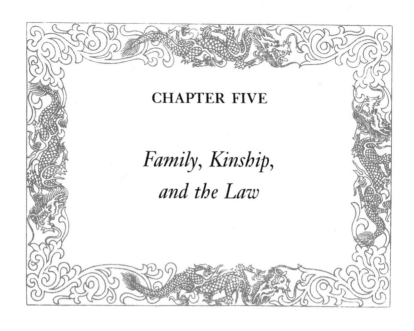

CHAPTER FIVE

Family, Kinship, and the Law

Intrafamily Homicide

IN 1697 THE BOARD OF PUNISHMENTS reviewed the following case: Liu Yuan, a native of Zhili, was beaten to death by his crazed wife, woman Zhang. The governor of Zhili tried the case under the statute "wife beating to death her husband" and sentenced Zhang to death by immediate decapitation. However, the Board of Punishments did not concur with the judgment of the governor. The board officials noted that the key issue in this case was the woman's illness. Although the Qing Code did not have any provisions for the offense of husband-killing due to a fit of madness, they held that the general principle of exempting insane offenders from punishment was applicable to insane women who killed their husbands. All insane persons lacked awareness of their actions, they insisted, and it should be of no consequence whether the perpetrator was a wife or not. The board ordered the governor of Zhili to reopen the case, with the specific charge to determine if the accused was genuinely mad.

The governor reported back that there was no doubt that Zhang was insane. Her neighbors had testified that she suffered from episodic bouts of madness. During one of these episodes, she burned all her clothes and took to the streets of the village, running and dancing wildly (classic symptoms of *kuang* madness). A local physician who had once ministered to her was able to verify to the local constables that her condition was incurable. By all accounts, it appeared that Zhang's illness was caused by some past provocation and since then, every time she was provoked to anger, her madness would return. The tragedy unfolded when Liu Yuan berated her son for some unknown reason. Zhang rose to her son's defense and started a shouting match with her husband. She became so agitated that she lost control of her senses and inflicted fatal blows on her husband with a piece of brick. She then turned her insane wrath on her son, and would have killed him too if a neighbor had not rushed to the lad's aid.

Having once again ascertained that woman Zhang was genuinely insane, and perhaps taking his cue from the Board of Punishments as well, the governor of Zhili changed his mind about the case and agreed with the board that the principle of exempting insane offenders from punishment was applicable to this case. The board upheld his revised opinion (*Li'an chuanji* 1722, 22:26a–26b).

The governor's earlier "mistake" was understandable. The relation between husband and wife was the third of the hallowed Three Bonds in the Confucian ethical system, which meant that when a woman (the inferior party) violated her husband's person she also violated the sacrosanct bond, an unforgivable offense. It was therefore natural for the governor to assume that insanity would not be allowed as a mitigating factor in this case. The fact that the Board of Punishments disagreed points to the powerful influence of the doctrine of mens rea. Had woman Zhang been pronounced sane, and therefore regarded as an intentional killer, her fate would have been very different. Traditional Chinese law was very harsh on women who did not fulfil their submissive wifely roles:

> In Ming and [Qing] the punishment for beating a husband was one hundred strokes regardless of whether he was injured or not, if he had accused her personally. If the beating resulted in a broken tooth, finger, toe, or rib, the punishment was increased three degrees; if permanent disability was caused, such as blindness or a broken limb, strangling was the punishment. If the assault resulted in death, the wife was beheaded immediately. (Ch'ü 1961, 106)

Even if it was found that the wife killed her husband by accident, the woman still was sentenced to death (ibid., 107). In stark contrast, the statutory punishment for "ordinary" accidental homicide was monetary redemption. Consider the following case from the *Xing'an huilan* as an illustration:

> [Li Erpan] loved his wife, Wang, very much. One evening, while Erpan was out, Wang went to bed because her knee pained her. About ten o'clock, her husband returned. He approached the bed in the dark and touched his wife. Half awake she kicked out, thinking that a stranger had entered the room. She struck Erpan in the belly. He then held her legs and demanded intercourse. Again she stretched her legs and she struck him in the belly. This time, he suffered great pain, stumbled, and died. Wang was sentenced to "immediate beheading," but a notation was made on [the governor's] report that her husband's death had been accidental. Her sentence was then reduced to "detention in prison for beheading." (ibid., 108)

Unlike their wives, husbands traditionally enjoyed a number of legal privileges. In Ming and Qing times, for example, a man could beat his wife without fearing prosecution, as long as he did not seriously injure her. Even then, if she elected not to press charges against him, he would not be held liable for the injury. Under Qing law, a man who was wounded by his wife had the right to divorce her without her consent, whereas a woman who was seriously wounded by her husband could not divorce him without first obtaining his assent. A man who beat his wife to death could not escape punishment, but the statutory sentence was strangulation, as opposed to beheading for a woman who killed her husband in a similar manner. However, husbands who killed their wives by accident were not held criminally liable (Ch'ü 1961, 105–107). Similarly, those who killed their wives in a fit of madness were not subject to punishment. The following case is an example:

One night in the autumn of 1730, Han Qiyun, a man with a three-year history of insanity, went berserk and hacked his wife to death with an axe. According to the governor's report, Han did not regain his senses after the incident but instead behaved in a crazy manner throughout the interrogations. He even made wild accusations about his deceased wife's marital infidelities. Although the officials were skeptical about his charges, they nonetheless summoned the dead woman's supposed paramours, Li and Deng, to court for questioning. Both men insisted that they were innocent, and their statements were corroborated by Han's son, his mother-in-law, and his brother-in-law. Having convinced himself that Han was genuinely insane, the governor applied the single homicide substatute of 1725 to the case and ordered Han to give his wife an elaborate burial. Additionally, for the sake of security, Han was to be locked up and kept under strict surveillance by his relatives.

This case took an inordinately long time to reach the Board of Punishments, and it was not until 1732 that board officials met to review it. The board did not find any fault with the governor's disposition of the case, but it did make explicit the point that since Han was the husband of the deceased there was no need to ask him to pay any burial compensation (*Cheng'an zhiyi* 1755, 19:41a–41b).

If we compare only the outcome of Han's case with that of woman Zhang's, it is difficult to say that Han enjoyed any preferential treatment because of his sex. However, if we compare the conduct of the two trials, we can see that Zhang was treated much more harshly by the provincial officials than Han was. Her illness was initially completely discounted as a mitigating factor and she was tried under the statute "wife beating to death her husband." Had not the Board of Punishments found fault with the provincial decision and ordered a reconsideration of the case, she might well have been executed. In contrast, Han was tried under the special substatute for single homicide committed by the insane, which automatically guaranteed very lenient treatment.

During a climate of great tolerance, it was perhaps not surprising that the Board of Punishments would consider madness a mitigating factor even in a crime as serious as "wife beating to death her husband." However, Zhang's case did not motivate the board to formulate a new substatute that would codify their decision in this particular case and guarantee clemency for women who killed their husbands in a fit of madness. For over one hundred more years, insane women who killed their husbands were dealt with on a case-by-case basis, and it is not known how many of the convicted women were as fortunate as Zhang. As the climate of opinion shifted in favor of more substantial punishment for all insane offenders, this arbitrary approach most probably spelled death for a number of women. The fairness of this approach was not questioned until 1806, when a particular case caught the attention of the Jiaqing emperor.

Woman Li began experiencing periodic fits of madness shortly after giving birth to a son in 1799. One evening in 1806, after the family had finished dinner, her husband retired early to bed but she stayed up to nurse her newborn daughter. She suddenly suffered another fit and, mistaking her sleeping husband for a black monster, bludgeoned him to death with an iron burner. She regained her senses soon afterwards and remained coherent in both thought and speech throughout the trial. The governor of Fengtian, who tried the case under the statute "wife beating to death her husband," found her guilty as charged and sentenced her to death by immediate decapitation. Both the Board of Punishments and the Grand Secretariat concurred with his judgment, and woman Li would have been executed had not the Jiaqing emperor interceded in her behalf.

Taking great interest in the case, the emperor studied the transcripts carefully and concluded that two mitigating factors should not be overlooked. First, Li was not, in his words, "in the habit of violating her husband" (*ping su ji wu ling fan*). Second, she was unquestionably insane. Citing as precedent a homicide case in Sichuan in which an insane man who killed his elder brother was given the reduced sentence of decapitation after the assizes (subsequently further reduced to life imprisonment) the emperor asked why wives were not accorded the same treatment as younger brothers. In the emperor's opinion, the degree of relationship between a wife and her husband was similar to that between brothers. He therefore ordered the Board of Punishments to review their files and to report to him how past cases were resolved.

The Board of Punishments reported back that the relationship between a wife and her husband was different from that between brothers. Whereas a wife had to observe three years of mourning for her husband, a younger brother had to observe only one year for his elder brother. It was therefore inappropriate to treat women who killed their husbands in the same manner as men who killed their elder brothers. The idea of giving Li the much-reduced sentence of life imprisonment was therefore opposed by the board. However, it was noted that records showed that in several instances guilty women did have their sentence of immediate beheading reduced one degree by the emperor. In other words, the board's position was that if the Jiaqing emperor so wished, he could reduce the woman's sentence by one degree, but his action should not be considered binding for future cases.

The emperor conceded that women who killed their husbands should be punished according to the stipulations of the appropriate laws. At the same time, however, he felt that women who were insane or who had never crossed their husbands could be treated more leniently. In an effort to reconcile the seriousness of the crime of husband-killing with his own feelings of compassion for women like Li, the Jiaqing emperor devised a five-step procedure for the handling of such cases: First, provincial officials were still to try such a case under the statute "wife beating to death her husband." They were then to forward the case on to the Board of Punishments for routine review. If the board did not find any fault with the provincial judgment, it would pass the case on to the Grand Secretariat. After a careful study of the transcripts, the Grand Secretariat was to write down its opinion, in the form of a memorandum, and send both the transcripts and the memorandum on to the Nine Chief Ministeries (*Jiuqing*, that is, the six boards plus the Court of Revision, the Censorate, and the Office of Transmission) for yet another round of review. The recommendation of the Nine Ministries would be forwarded to the emperor, who would make the final decision. As for this particular case, the Jiaqing emperor reduced woman Li's sentence by one degree, thereby giving her the benefit of having her conviction reviewed again at the Autumn Assizes (*Jiaqing shilu* 1964, 2415–16; 2424–25; *Xing'an huilan* 1968, 2123).

It is important to note that Jiaqing's intervention in this case and the five-step procedure that resulted from it did not lead to the formulation of a new substatute. As was mentioned in Chapter One, although imperial edicts of the sort just described did have the effect of formal law in the sense that they were supposed to be binding on future decisions, until they became substatutes many judicial officials appeared uncertain about their applicability. Among the innovations relating to insane criminals this procedure was the only one that failed to evolve into a substatute. All others acquired that status, albeit in some instances in vastly modified form. Nonetheless, it appears that the edict did heighten the sensitivity of provincial officials to the mitigating factor of insanity. The following case offers an example of this new awareness.

In 1812, the governor of Anhui submitted a memorial to the Board of Punishments concerning the case of woman Zhang, who strangled her husband during a fit of madness and burned his remains. According to testimony provided by the local constable, neighbors, and the victim's son and elder brother, Zhang suffered from recurring bouts of madness, a claim that was supported by a physician who was called in by the officials to examine the accused (this is one of the rare instances in which officials consulted a physician). The Board of Punishment agreed that Zhang's illness was well documented. They made a special note that since she lived in a very remote and deserted location, if she had schemed to kill her husband she could easily have disposed of his body and destroyed all evidence. The fact that she left her husband's charred remains in the kitchen, where they could easily be discovered, pointed to the fact that she did not commit premeditated murder. The board upheld the governor's judgment (*Xing'an huilan* 1968, 2123). It is noteworthy that, in contrast to the position taken by his counterparts in the cases presented above, the governor of Anhui accepted insanity as a relevant and significant fact in this case.

How did Li (and others like her who benefitted from the Jiaqing procedure) fare compared to "ordinary" insane killers? Readers may recall that in 1802 the Board of Punishments classified insane murderers into two categories: those who were previously registered and therefore indisputably insane, and those who were not registered but had managed to obtain statements from their victim's family that confirmed their illness. The stipulated punishment for the first category was life imprisonment, and that for the second category was strangulation after the assizes. Criminals who claimed to have become suddenly insane, but could not obtain corroborating statements from their victim's family, were sentenced to decapitation after the assizes. It is apparent that, although the Jiaqing emperor felt sympathy for Li, the best he could do was to reduce the sentence of immediate decapitation by one degree to decapitation after the assizes, which was the same punishment as that for killers who were deemed sane by the authorities. It is obvious that the principle of aggravation had taken precedent over the principle of clemency.

The difference between the disposition of Li's case (1806) and that of Zhang (1697) shows clearly how the juridical climate had changed for the criminally insane. But Li was more than a casualty of the hardening attitude; she was also a victim of legal discrimination against women. Consider, in contrast, the following almost-contemporaneous case involving the killing of a woman by her insane husband:

In 1813, Zheng Wenhuan, a native of Sichuan province, was arrested for killing his wife. At the time of his apprehension, as well as throughout the entire interrogation process, Zheng exhibited many of the classic symptoms of madness. He appeared wide-eyed and confused, and the interrogators could not understand him. The governor-general of Sichuan was convinced that Zheng was genuinely insane. He consulted the Qing Code and decided that two laws in particular were applicable to the case in question: the single-homicide substatute for insane murderers and the statute governing the accidental killing of a woman by her husband. The former law stipulated life-imprisonment while the latter excused the husband of any criminal liability. Citing both laws in his resolution of the case, the governor-general excused Zheng for the murder of his wife, but he also sentenced him to life imprisonment. The Board of Punishments concurred with his decision (*Xing'an huilan* 1968, 2120).

The difference between the treatment of Zheng and that of Li is obvious. Whereas Li was given the sentence of decapitation after the assizes, Zheng was declared not criminally liable for the death of his wife. Although he was given a life sentence, it was purely for the sake of public security and was not intended to be punishment for killing his wife. The inequity was, as noted earlier, deeply rooted in the hierarchical structure of the traditional Chinese family and the legal system that reinforced such a structure. Juniors (wives, children, daughters-in-law, nieces, nephews, and younger brothers and sisters) who violated the person of their seniors invariably had to pay heavily for having done so.

In 1713 the governor of Jiangsu reported to the Board of Punishments that woman Jiang was arrested for beating to death her mother-in-law, woman Xie. Jiang had a long history of madness; in fact, she had been kept in a locked room in the family home. One day during the autumn of 1711, Xie thought to herself that her daughter-in-law appeared to have recovered somewhat from her illness and decided to unchain the younger woman for a short while. Knowing that her son would oppose such an action, she sent him out of the house on the pretext that the crops needed to be harvested. Unfortunately, Jiang suddenly suffered a fit of madness and clubbed her mother-in-law to death. She was arrested and brought to trial. The provincial officials did not doubt that she was genuinely mad, but during the early phase of their deliberations they decided that her illness should not be taken as a mitigating factor and that such being the case, her just punishment would be *lingchi*. However, when they consulted the casebooks, they came across the woman Zhang case (1697, presented earlier in this chapter), which indicated to them that clemency might be given to Jiang as well. The governor of Jiangsu made a notation about the parallels between the two cases in his report to the Board of Punishments.

However, the board ruled that the two cases represented very different situations. Whereas Zhang killed her husband, Jiang killed her mother-in-law. Even though in the *wufu* system of mourning a woman observed the same degree of mourning (first degree) for her husband and mother-in-law, the board ruled that the latter was a more grievous offense. Such being the case, it would be inappropriate to accord Jiang the same treatment as that given Zhang. They ruled that the statute "woman beating to death the parents of her husband" should be applied to the case and that Jiang be given the statutory sentence of *lingchi*. In other words, they did not allow the woman's illness to be a mitigating factor. They then presented their decision to the Kangxi emperor for his adjudication.

Kangxi took a more moderate stance than had the Board of Punishments. He noted several pertinent facts: Jiang had a long history of madness; her mother-in-law personally unlocked her chains; and it was during the fit suffered at the moment she regained her freedom that she clubbed her mother-in-law to death. Taking these circumstances into account, Kangxi ruled that Jiang should be given clemency and spared the ultimate punishment of *lingchi*. He felt that a more appropriate sentence was decapitation after the assizes. He also ruled that since Jiang's husband was at work in the fields at the time of the incident and was not at all aware of the goings on, he should not be held responsible for her offense (*Cheng'an zhiyi* 1755, 19:39a–39b).

This case illustrates very clearly the construction of hierarchy and power within the family, especially with respect to women. The decision to deny Jiang the same clemency accorded Zhang points to the fact that the power differential between mother-in-law and daughter-in-law was greater than that between husband and wife.

In 1756, the Board of Punishments reviewed a case of fratricide involving an insane man. The governor of Zhejiang reported that he had sentenced to death by immediate decapitation a certain Gong Yuan, who killed his brother during a fit of madness. In the same document the governor also noted that he had come across in his research an earlier fratricide case in which the insane offender was given the reduced sentence of decapitation after the assizes, and for this reason he recommended to the Board of Punishments a similar judgment. The board, however, ruled that Gong should not have his death penalty reduced and presented its ruling to the Qianlong emperor. The emperor subsequently referred the case to the Nine Chief Ministries for their evaluation.

The opinion written by the Nine Chief Ministries included a summary of the particulars of the case, to wit: Gong Yuan had a long history of madness. In 1755 the local magistrate ordered both his elder brother, Gong Hua, and the local constable to keep a close watch over him. In compliance with the order, Gong Hua took custody of his younger brother and locked him up in their clan's ancestral hall. One month into his confinement, while his aunt was paying him a visit, Gong Yuan begged her to set him free. The aunt, seeing that her nephew's condition seemed to have improved somewhat, thereupon unchained him.

For a month or two, everything seemed to go well. Although Gong found an outside job, he preferred to stay in close touch with his family, spending an occasional night or two at his aunt's house. During these visits, he shared the bed with his elder brother. One evening he found his brother lying ill in bed. After exchanging pleasantries with him, Gong Yuan noticed a firewood ax next to the bed. This somehow triggered a sudden fit of madness. He picked up the ax and hacked his brother several times, killing him instantly. Such were the details of the case as known to the Nine Chief Ministries. They concluded that the homicide was occasioned by the ill-considered decision of the aunt to free Gong Yuan from his confinement. Because they were convinced that the offender was genuinely insane, they ruled that his offense was different from "ordinary" cases of fratricide and recommended that his sentence be reduced by one degree to decapitation after the assizes. The Qianlong emperor accepted their recommendation (*Cheng'an xinpian* 1763, 9:21a–22b). Although Gong Yuan was ultimately granted a lesser death sentence, his sentence could have been even lighter. The following case serves as a contrast:

In 1796 the Board of Punishments reviewed a trial report submitted by the governor of Hunan concerning Liu Zumiao, who killed his younger brother during a fit of madness. He was arrested but died in prison while awaiting sentencing. The governor proposed to apply to the case the statute "elder brother killing younger brother in an accident," which would acquit Liu posthumously of all criminal liability. The Board of Punishments, however, ruled that the most appropriate law for the case in question was the 1762 substatute for insane homicide. They explained that although the penalty for both accidental homicide and insane homicide was payment of a burial indemnity of 12.42 taels of silver, the two offenses should not be considered analogous. For whereas the accidental killer would be set free after payment of indemnity, such freedom was not allowed an insane slayer. As for the case at hand, the board ruled that had Liu not died in prison while waiting to be sentenced, he would have been given the statutory sentence of life imprisonment; no burial indemnity would have to be collected because his victim was a younger brother (*Xing'an huilan* 1968, 2119–2120). We can see in these two cases how birth order translated into a difference between life and death.

In 1784, Liu Jinliang, a native of Shandong province, became afflicted with madness. Because he appeared to be harmless, his relatives did not report his illness to the authorities, nor did anyone maintain a close watch over him. One summer day in 1785, while he was cutting grass in his father's fields, he suffered a relapse of his illness, but no one paid any particular attention to him. This nonchalant attitude toward his condition ultimately resulted in tragedy, because in the middle of that night, Liu became raving mad and slit the throat of his grandfather's cousin, a *sima* (fifth-degree) relative, with a sickle. Fortunately, his father managed to wrest the sickle from his hands and eventually subdued him, averting a potential massacre.

Liu did not regain his senses but remained completely incoherent throughout the interrogation process. Although the officials could not extract any sense or information out of him, they were able to obtain statements from his neighbors, the local constable, and the victim's son, all of whom agreed that Liu was genuinely insane and that there was no reason to suspect that he had any motive for killing his uncle. Before he could conclude the case, however, the governor of Shandong had to decide whether the principle of aggravation was applicable to the case. In the end, he reasoned that, because the victim was only a fifth-degree relative, there was no need to give Liu an aggravated sentence. He thus sentenced Liu to life imprisonment and ordered him to pay the victim's family 12.42 taels of silver.

The Board of Punishments, however, found fault with the governor's ruling. The officials who reviewed the case disagreed with his assessment that the *sima* relationship between Liu and his grandfather's cousin was too insignificant to warrant an aggravated sentence. They maintained that, although *sima* was a minor mourning degree, it still described a relationship that was based on common ancestry (*tongzong*). Therefore, it was improper to discount it as the governor had done in this case. The board ordered the governor to reconsider his decision and, particularly, to take into account the gravity of killing a senior relative. The governor took his cue and changed the sentence from life imprisonment to decapitation after the assizes, a punishment that befitted one who had killed his senior (*Boan xinpian* 1968, 1783–89).

This case firmly established the precedent for invoking the principle of aggravation in cases involving mourning-degree relatives, regardless of how low the degree of relationship might be. For example, in 1792, a Sichuan man was sentenced to decapitation after the assizes for killing his mother-in-law, a *sima* senior by marriage. The governor-general of Sichuan had originally given him only a life sentence, but the Board of Punishments, citing the Liu Jinliang precedent, ordered him to change his ruling to reflect the gravity of killing a senior relative (*Xing'an huilan* 1968, 2120). Once again, the principle of clemency was modified by the principle of aggravation.

We have seen from the examples presented so far that the *wufu* or "five mourning degrees" system was crucial to the determination of degree of criminal responsibility. If the victim was a senior relative, guilt was aggravated, but if the victim was a junior relative, it was mitigated. So far, we have looked only at single homicides. Would the special legal privileges enjoyed by a superordinate be neutralized in cases of multiple homicide where the victims were junior relations? Would the grievous nature of multiple homicide negate the status differential between perpetrator and victims? How would the government respond to multiple homicide committed by an insane person against senior relatives?

In 1814, the Statutes Commission drafted a memorandum after officials had reviewed an intrafamily multiple homicide case. The document began with a presentation of relevant laws:

> According to the existing law governing the crime of killing three members of the same family, if all three victims were junior relatives of the offender, but one of them was a mourning-degree relative, the homicide should be treated as though the murderer and his victims were of equal status. The criminal

should therefore be sentenced to immediate decapitation and exposure of his head. According to another substatute, an insane person who killed two or more members of the same family should be sentenced to strangulation after the assizes. Also, [according to another substatute] an insane murderer who recovered sufficiently to give coherent testimony should be given the same sentence as one who killed another during an affray. Additionally, according to the relevant statutes an uncle who beat to death his nephew is liable to one hundred blows with heavy bamboo and three years of penal servitude, but a man who beat to death the wife of his younger brother is liable to the same penalty as one who killed another person of the same status. Finally, the statutory sentence for homicide committed during an affray is strangulation after the assizes. (*Lüliguan shuotie* 1805–1814, no pagination)

Having cited the laws they considered to be relevant to the case in question, the Statutes Commission proceeded next to render their interpretation of the laws. They understood the sentence of immediate decapitation and exposure of the head to be applicable only to *premeditated* multiple homicide. They noted that the statutory punishment for multiple homicide committed by an insane person was strangulation after the assizes and that the lighter sentence was an acknowledgment that insane persons lacked awareness of their actions. Thus, even if they could testify coherently afterwards, they still could not be tried under the regular statute for premeditated murder. As for the crime of killing three junior relatives, one of whom was a mourning-degree relative, the commission noted that there were no specific laws in the Qing Code that dealt with such a situation. However, they believed that there were precedents established to suggest that the case could be adjudicated as though the slayer and victim were of equal status.

The case that generated this review of relevant laws involved a multiple homicide committed by Chen Changzhi, an insane man. His victims were the wife of his younger brother and her son and daughter. At the conclusion of the provincial-level trial, Chen was sentenced to immediate decapitation and exposure of his head in public, the governor having applied the regular statute for premeditated multiple homicide in which the victims were not of the same family. The Statutes Commission ultimately disagreed with the provincial judgment. They ruled that because Chen was able to give a coherent statement after his arrest, this aspect of the case could be covered by the substatute of 1806, which stipulated a sentence of strangulation after the assizes. Since his nephew and niece were junior relatives, his sentence for their murders should be only penal servitude. As for the murder of his sister-in-law, because it was committed in the course of a multiple homicide, statutory provisions required that it be treated as single homicide in which the slayer and victim were of the same status. Accordingly, they ruled, his punishment should be strangulation after the assizes (*Lüliguan shuotie* 1805–1814, no pagination).

We can glean from the deliberations recorded in the case above the fine distinctions in familial relationships. For example, the difference between the penalty for an uncle who has beat to death his nephew and that for a man who has killed the wife of his younger brother reflects the difference in status within the *wufu* system. Within this construct, an uncle is a second-degree (*zicui*) relation whereas a sister-in-law is third-degree (*dagong*). It is interesting that the Statutes Commission did not make specific reference to the landmark 1776 insane multiple homicide substatute, which stipulated a sentence of strangulation after the assizes; however, their logical process ultimately led to the same outcome as far as sentencing was concerned. If they had chosen to apply the 1776 substatute to the case, it would still have required their conclusion that the case be adjudicated as homicide involving parties of equal status.

In 1817, the Board of Punishments reviewed the case of Li Dakuei, who in a fit of madness killed his wife and his uncle (a second-degree relative), and wounded his aunt (second-degree) and three other members of his extended family. The governor of Henan was satisfied that Li was genuinely insane and that the rampage was caused by his illness. However, because one of his victims was his uncle, a senior relative, the governor decided that Li could not be tried under the substatutes governing homicides committed by the insane; rather he should be tried according to the statute governing the offense of a junior beating to death a senior relative, which stipulated a sentence of immediate decapitation. In his memorial to the Board of Punishments, the governor noted that because of the grievous nature of Li's transgression there was no need to include an insert regarding Li's illness. (Such inserts were usually submitted to call attention to mitigating circumstances so the board officials could decide whether to reduce the recommended sentence.)

The officials at the Board of Punishments disagreed with the governor's decision not to submit an insert with his memorial. They had gone over old records and discovered two earlier cases which could be regarded as precedents. In 1799, in the province of Shandong, Wang Bingru was originally sentenced to immediate decapitation for having killed his aunt and a kitchen hand during a fit of madness. A special insert describing his illness was included in the provincial report to the Board of Punishments, and his sentence was subsequently reduced by one degree to decapitation after the assizes. In 1812, again in the province of Shandong, Wang Shuqin was originally sentenced to immediate decapitation for having killed five children during a fit of madness. The Board of Punishments subsequently reduced his sentence to strangulation after the assizes. Both criminals were deemed "deserving of punishment" at the Autumn Assizes, but they escaped execution because, electing to save their lives, the Jiaqing emperor did not put a check against their names.

In the opinion of the Board of Punishments, the case being reviewed was similar to the Wang Bingru case as far as the number of lives taken was concerned, but because an additional four persons were injured during the rampage, the case should be regarded as more grievous. Ultimately, however, the board downplayed the number of victims involved, because in their opinion insane persons could not know the identities or number of the people they were wounding. The critical point to be considered was that in *all* cases of homicide committed by the insane, the slayers did not know what they were doing. It was only proper that appropriate judicial procedures established for such cases should be universally followed and that reports on these cases should all include an insert noting the illness of the offender. The summary of this case as it appeared in the *Xing'an huilan* contained no other details, but a notation appended at the end did mention that an insert was included in a subsequent memorial to the Nine Chief Ministries and that Li's sentence was eventually reduced to decapitation after the assizes (*Xing'an huilan* 1968, 2122). In other words, insanity was allowed as a mitigating factor. If we compare this case to that of Chen Changzhi (whose victims were junior relations), in which Chen was given the sentence of strangulation after the assizes, we can see that the principle of aggravation was applied here.

Since the Chinese kinship network was so complex and the *wufu* system so vast, it was not always easy for judicial officials to figure out precise degrees of relationship. For example, in 1843 the Jiangsu department of the Board of Punishments considered the case of Wang Yulong, a resident of Jiangsu province, who was charged with killing woman Tan during a fit of madness. This was not a routine case, because the relationship between Wang and his victim was extremely complex.

Wang Yulong's great-grandfather had four sons. The eldest, Zhangtai, was Yulong's grandfather. The second son was Xitai. The third son, Yintai, was married to Tan. Because the couple did not have any sons, they adopted Yulong's natural father as heir. The fourth son, Kuitai, had one son, Jingxi. Because he had no sons of his own, Jingxi adopted Yulong to be his heir. In other words, Yulong's adoptive father was a first cousin of his natural father, and his natural father's adoptive mother was Tan, who herself was the aunt (by marriage) of Yulong's adoptive father.

The governor of Jiangsu found himself in a judicial maze. By one way of reckoning, Tan was only the aunt of Yulong's adoptive father, which would make her a *xiaogong* (fourth-degree) senior. The crime of beating to death a *xiaogong* elder was, according to the relevant statute, punishable by decapitation. Reckoned differently, however, Tan might be considered equivalent to Yulong's grandmother. After all, the governor reasoned, she was the adoptive mother of Yulong's natural father. Should not his punishment be *lingchi*, the statutory sentence for someone who killed his grandparent? At the same time, however, the fact that Tan was not Yulong's natural grandmother should not be ignored, because it meant that his indebtedness or degree of obligation toward Tan was not the same as that toward his natural grandmother. The sentence of *lingchi*, in this case, might be excessive. Unable to resolve this knotty problem, the governor turned to the Board of Punishments for guidance.

The officials at the Board of Punishments were unable to offer the governor immediate advice, because the Qing Code contained no provisions for an offense involving a familial relationship as complicated as that in the case being considered. They turned instead to the Board of Rites for help. Surely, the judicial officials reasoned, the experts on matters dealing with propriety should be able to define precisely the relationship between Yulong and Tan. The Rites officials, however, found themselves stumped, because they, too, could not find any precedents or regulations that were appropriate to this particular situation. It was thus up to the Board of Punishments to decide on the matter. After much deliberation, board officials wrote the following:

> The reason why a person who violates his grandmother is always sentenced according to the regular statutes for the particular offense, with no mitigating circumstances allowed, is that he has done harm to someone he is directly descended from.
>
> In this particular case, the victim was the adoptive mother of the offender's natural father, thus it can be said that a kinship relationship between the two exists and cannot be lightly dismissed. Since the offender has been adopted into another agnate line, he is now bound by another set of kinship ties and the

old bond between him and his natural father's adoptive mother—
that is, as grandson and grandmother—is no longer relevant. In
any case, their present relationship is—and has to be—different from that which binds a grandparent and grandchild in the
same agnate line.

The point has been made that since the deceased was the
adoptive mother of the offender's natural father, a [very close]
mourning-degree relationship exists between the two that must
not be slighted. [However, there is another way to look at the
relationship.] If we consider only the present kinship tie between the two, the deceased, being the offender's adoptive father's aunt, would be his senior relative and he could be punished according to the relevant substatute for the offense of
beating to death a *xiaogong* senior. [Even if we opt for this defi-
nition, we would be acknowledging a mourning-degree relationship between the two.]

However, we have here only very sketchy information from
the governor to work with. The facts of the case are so uncertain that it is difficult to make a decision. The governor should
thoroughly investigate the case and submit the pertinent information, along with his recommendations, to the board. We will
decide on the merits of the case at that time, [when we have
more information].

Unable to render a decision regarding the precise relationship
between Wang Yulong and Tan, the Board of Punishments
employed a face-saving move and passed the buck back to the
governor. The ultimate fate of Wang Yulong is unknown
(*Xing'an huilan xupian* 1970, 3965–68).

Two years later, in 1845 (the next scheduled opportunity to
enact new substatutes), the government formulated a substatute that dealt specifically with cases involving *qigong* (sec-
ond- and third-degree) relatives. This substatute, a complicated and comprehensive law, is a fine example of the Qing
legalistic mind at work:

He who, during a fit of madness, takes the life of his *qigong* senior; or the life of a senior plus that of a member of the senior's
household who is the killer's junior, and for whose death he is
not criminally liable; or the life of a senior plus that of another,
unrelated person, is to be sentenced to death by immediate de-

capitation. However, it is possible in the above cases for the judicial officials to submit a request to the emperor asking for clemency.

> He who takes the lives of two *qigong* seniors, whether or not they belong in the same household; or the life of one senior plus that of a member of the senior's household who is the killer's junior, and for whose death he is liable to the penalty of strangulation; or the life of a senior, plus the lives of two other, unrelated persons, shall be sentenced to death by immediate decapitation. A petition for reduction of sentence is not permitted in said cases. (Nakamura 1973, 197)

Although there appears to be no particular case or communication that contributed directly to this new substatute, it is possible that the complicated and perhaps unresolved Wang Yulong case convinced board officials that a more specific law governing intrafamily homicide was long overdue.

Filial Obligations

It was noted in Chapter Three that successive dynastic codes specified harsh punishments for unfilial conduct. The various codes reinforced the virtue of filial piety in another, and more positive, way. The principle of *liuyang chengsi*, for example, allowed a criminal to have his sentence suspended or even pardoned if he was the sole support of his aged parents. The earliest case of a criminal having his death sentence commuted because his aged parents needed care was in A.D. 327 when Emperor Cheng (326–342) pardoned a condemned official, Kong Hui, because he was an only son. T'ung-tsu Ch'ü details the evolution of this principle:

> The earliest legal regulation of this sort was formulated in the Northern Wei dynasty. Under it, cases in which the criminal's grandparents or parents were over seventy and had no adult children or other first-degree side-line relatives to take care of them could be presented to the emperor for special consideration.
>
> Since the time of [Tang] this idea has been the pattern followed and similar regulations were inserted in the codes of the various dynasties. In [Tang, Song, Yuan, Ming, and Qing] law, a criminal who had been sentenced to death for a crime that

was not unpardonable, and whose grandparents or parents were old or were suffering from a serious illness that required care, and who had no adult male members in the family, could ask that his case be given special consideration. Final disposition rested with the emperor. . . .
    Widowed mothers were specially dealt with. In usual cases, according to [Qing] law, a criminal's parent had to be over seventy before his case could be appealed, but if his mother was a widow, no age limit was set. All that was demanded was that the mother had been a widow for twenty years. . . . Such merciful treatment was shown her because it was believed that it was difficult for a widow to bring up her son. (Ch'ü 1961, 76–77)

The antiquity of the principle of *liuyang chengsi* did not mean that it was so well established and familiar that there was no room for disagreement or misunderstanding. We find in the *Veritable Records of the Qianlong emperor* a fascinating discourse on the subject:

In 1740, the censor Liu Fang'ai submitted a memorial to the emperor concerning the formulation of a new regulation governing *liuyang chengsi* that would be applied to criminals who had been condemned to death for murdering their elder brothers. He suggested that these criminals be allowed to return home on a term basis, provided that a bonded statement could be obtained from their clan elders and neighbors, guaranteeing their good behavior. After such a criminal had served his aged parents and fathered a son as well, he would be returned to prison to serve out his sentence.

The Board of Punishments opposed Liu's recommendation. Board officials cited a decision that was arrived at only a year earlier, in 1739, concerning a fratricide case in Shanxi. In his disposition of this particular case, the governor of Shanxi, following standard practice, sentenced the murderer (the younger brother of the deceased), Xu Zhi, to immediate decapitation, but he also included in his report a petition for clemency to the Qianlong emperor on the grounds that Xu's parents were aged and had no other sons to serve them. As a consequence of the appeal, the emperor reduced Xu's sentence to detention in prison to await execution, thereby in effect sparing his life.

The Board of Punishments noted that the emperor also issued an order to the effect that all subsequent cases of this kind should be dealt with in like manner. In other words, in the board's opinion, the issue had already been resolved. The emperor was not impressed with the board's presentation. He noted that a criminal who murdered his elder brother deserved the penalty of immediate decapitation. If he happened to be the last surviving son of his aged parents, he could petition for clemency on the grounds that his parents needed his care. That he could do so was an example of extralegal benevolence. The emperor added that the criminal must not be let off too lightly. This was why, in the Xu Zhi case, he did not pardon the criminal outright, but instead reduced his sentence to detention in prison to await execution.

The emperor went on to say that both the censor and the Board of Punishments had failed to take note that, when he reduced Xu's sentence, he also issued an edict stating that in the future criminals in the same situation should be kept in prison for two to three years, during which time they would have the opportunity to reflect on their crime and repent. When they had done so, they could be released from prison to serve their parents. The emperor pointedly noted that the censor's memorial and the board's refutation showed that both sides had failed to understand the full meaning of his earlier actions. He ordered the Nine Chief Ministries to study the matter carefully and present their findings to him at a later date (*Qianglong shilu* 1964, 1836).

Bodde and Morris note that in 1769 it was decided that criminals who were the sole heirs of *deceased* parents could also be released from prison to continue the family sacrifices to the ancestors (1973, 41). These requests, however, were not automatically granted, as the following case shows:

In 1818, the governor of Jiangsu province submitted a memorial to the Jiaqing emperor requesting permission to release from jail Hua Fengbao, an insane prisoner who was serving a life sentence for killing his neighbor. The reason for the petition was to allow Hua to return home to continue family sacrifices to his ancestors. The emperor sent the case to the

Statutes Commission for study. Specifically, the question was whether convicted insane murderers, other than those who killed their wives, could be released from prison in order to continue ancestral sacrifices. He also instructed the commission to add the appropriate notations to the Qing Code at the time of the next round of revisions. (Note: As was pointed out in Chapter Three, a husband who killed his wife in a fit of madness was not held criminally liable for the act. He was imprisoned only because he might still be a threat to public well-being; he was not serving a prison term per se. Such being the case, his recovery from insanity, once certified, would be sufficient to allow him to return home to serve his parent[s] or to continue family sacrifices.)

The Statutes Commission recommended rejection of the petition. Their decision was based on two relevant substatutes. The first, enacted in 1801, stipulated that a killer who had recovered from insanity could petition for his release from prison in order to take care of his aged parents. The commissioners pointed out, however, that this applied only to criminals who remained insane after the homicide and whose recovery took place while they were serving their life term. (Note: This law also placed the burden of surveillance and control squarely on the shoulders of local officials as well as the former inmate's relatives. Additionally, it stipulated that, should the repatriated criminal suffer a relapse and cause trouble again, he would be remanded to jail, never to be set free again [Xue 1970, 861].)

The second law, formulated in 1814, extended eligibility to include those who regained sanity shortly after their apprehension. But in order to be eligible, they must have already served five years in prison. The substatute of 1814 also made it possible for an only son whose parents were deceased to request commutation of sentence, but only if he was imprisoned for killing his wife in a fit of madness. The Statutes Commission pointed out that because the intent of the 1814 law was to provide more prisoners with the opportunity for commutation, the five-year prerequisite was absolutely necessary if the cunning designs of hardened criminals were to be thwarted.

As for the case in question, the commission was of the opinion that Hua did not meet the conditions set down by the 1814 substatute. More significantly, the commission pointed out that in their opinion, the real purpose of the use of *chengsi* was to spare a criminal's life; to say that he was spared so that he could continue family sacrifices was only a pretext. After all, the commission noted, whereas aged parents could be properly taken care of only by their biological sons, ancestral sacrifices could be continued via a number of means. (Adoption would be one alternative.) Therefore, a prisoner whose parents were old and had no other sons to serve them had a very good reason to petition for release from prison, but one whose parents were deceased did not (*Xing'an huilan* 1968, 2117–18).

The substatutes of 1801 and 1814, formulated to deal specifically with petitions from the criminally insane, are a good measure of the Qing government's attempts to reconcile state sponsorship of filial piety with the need to protect society from the danger posed by insane persons. The government did not want to deprive aged and helpless parents of the filial care that was due them from their sons, but it was reluctant to set free prisoners who had proven themselves to be uncontrollably murderous. The following three cases illustrate the laws in action. In the first case the petitioner did not have the benefit of the substatute of 1814 and consequently suffered because of it.

In 1809 the Zhili department of the Board of Punishments considered a request by inmate Liang Liu for permission to be released from prison so he could take care of his aged mother. After some deliberation, the officials drafted the following memorandum:

> According to the substatute [of 1806], in cases of homicide committed because of insanity, if upon examination it was determined that the offender had not regained his or her senses, the sentence should be life imprisonment. If the onset of the illness was very sudden, but subsequently he or she recovered and could provide coherent testimony during the trial, the substatute stipulated that if a corroborating statement could be obtained from the victim's family, the offender should be sen-

tenced by analogy to the statute governing homicide committed during an affray.

Also, an insane [male] killer sentenced to life imprisonment
may, on the grounds that his parents are old and do not have
other sons to care for them, be eligible for consideration to
have his prison sentence commuted, so that he may return
home to care for his parents and continue ancestral sacrifices.
However, his request will be considered only if he has fully recovered from his illness and the local authorities have certified
this fact in the form of a bonded statement. [We see again that
physicians were not included in the certification process.]

In the case of homicide committed during an affray [which is
a less grievous offense than premeditated murder], the convicted criminal, even though he did not request commutation
of his death sentence at the time of conviction—because his
parents were not considered aged—may at a later time, when
circumstances have changed, request to have his sentence commuted on the grounds of *liuyang chengsi*. However, the provincial officials must first ascertain that his death sentence has been
reprieved at the Autumn Assizes and that his grandparents or
parents are truly aged, or that his widowed mother has remained chaste for a long time. If the said conditions are met,
the governor can then send the request to the Board of Punishments for consideration.

The policy outlined above is applicable also to prisoners convicted of the crime of homicide committed during a fit of madness who are currently serving life sentences. But they must already have spent many years in prison and have been certified
as having fully recovered from their illness. As for those who
regained their senses shortly after the homicide and could testify coherently during the trial, the policy has been to sentence
them to death. [This policy was instituted] because of the concern that some murderers might feign madness [in order to escape punishment]. It has been the government's policy to deny
this category of criminals the privilege to request commutation
of their sentences on the grounds of *liuyang chengsi* in spite of
the fact that, at the time of the Autumn Assizes, it was known
that their parents were old and had no other sons to care for
them. Those criminals [whose circumstances did not meet the
conditions set by the *liuyang chengsi* substatutes] at the time of
the Autumn Assizes, but who subsequently found themselves

[with aged parents who needed care], also had not been allowed the privilege of *liuyang chengsi*.

In this particular case, the inmate Liang Liu because of insanity killed his wife and son. He regained his senses shortly afterwards and was able to testify coherently during the trial. He was sentenced, according to the statute "husband beating to death his wife," to strangulation after the assizes. [Note: It is likely that the regular statute was applied to this case, instead of the insanity substatute, because it involved multiple deaths. The summary was unclear about this point.] His death sentence had been reprieved twice.

The governor-general has submitted a memorial on behalf on Liang Liu, requesting permission to release him on the grounds of *liuyang chengsi*. He reports that the said criminal confessed during the trial that his father had been dead for more than eighteen years, that his mother was over sixty years old, and that he had one surviving son. The governor-general adds that he has now ascertained that Liang's mother has remained a widow for more than twenty years, that Liang's son is now thirteen years old, and that the Liang household does not have any adult male.

In light of the laws and precedents [cited above], this department has decided that the governor-general's request [on behalf of Liang] should be denied. (*Shuotie leipian* 1835, 2:18a–19a)

In 1845 the governor of Henan forwarded a petition to the Board of Punishments to release a prisoner, Gao Hu, from jail so he could serve his aged mother. Gao had been sentenced to death in 1825 for killing his *xiaogong* uncle (a fourth-degree relative) in a fit of madness. The original sentence was immediate decapitation, but the Daoguang emperor, acting upon the recommendation of the Nine Ministries, reduced it to decapitation after the assizes. During the Autumn Assizes, Gao was found "deserving of punishment," but fortunately for him, the emperor instead further reduced his sentence to life imprisonment. At the time of the petition Gao had already spent twenty years in prison.

The Board of Punishments, after some deliberation, recommended to the emperor approval of Gao's petition. A number of factors figured in the favorable recommendation. First of all, it was determined to the officials' satisfaction that Gao had completely recovered from his illness. This was an important consideration. Second, Gao had already spent at least twenty years in prison, far longer than the five-year requirement stipulated by the 1814 substatute. Third, Gao's mother was over seventy years old and had been a widow for over forty years, and Gao Hu was her only son. (The trial summary did not explain why she waited so long to ask for her son's release. It might be that Gao had not recovered from his illness until very recently.) Fourth, the victim was not an only son. Fifth, the victim's three sons supported Gao's petition for clemency. The emperor agreed with the Board of Punishments. Following established regulations, Gao was ordered to wear a cangue for two months and after receiving a "reprimand" (*ze*, perhaps a euphemism for "beating" here), was released from prison to take care of his aged mother (*Xing'an huilan xupian* 1970, 275–76).

In 1821, Feng Jinjong, a native of Zhili, was found guilty of killing an unrelated person in a fit of madness. In accordance with the 1806 single-homicide substatute, Feng was given the sentence of strangulation after the assizes (he regained his senses after the homicide). At the time of sentencing, it was specifically noted that because Feng's parents were old and needed his care, he could be released after he had spent five years in prison.

His death sentence was reprieved at the Autumn Assizes, and in 1826, after Feng had served five years of his prison term, the governor-general of Zhili took up the case for consideration. At the time, because he learnt that Feng had been suffering from episodic bouts of madness, he did not process Feng's release. However, three years later, in 1829, having determined that Feng had fully recovered, the governor-general submitted a memorial to the Board of Punishments requesting commutation of Feng's sentence so that he could return home to care for his aged parents. He noted that Feng's father was in his eighties and his mother was in her late seventies. They had no other adult male to take care of them. The governor-general also pointed out that Feng's victim was not an only son. The Board of Punishments ruled against the petition for immediate release, noting that because Feng's recovery was relatively recent, he had failed to meet the five-year requirement. They instructed the governor-general to determine the precise date of Feng's recovery. Five full years after that date, provided that he had not suffered a relapse during the period, Feng's petition could be considered again (ibid., 1970, 317–18).

Since only sons could continue family sacrifices to ancestors, and daughters (married or unmarried) were not counted on to take care of their aged parents, the principle of *liuyang chengsi* benefitted only men. The denial to women of two reasons for requesting commutation of prison sentences struck some officials as patently unfair. One of them, the governor of Anhui, tried in 1840 to rectify this inequity. The governor had taken an interest in the fate of woman Wang, a prisoner who had already served two years of her life sentence for killing a retainer during a fit of madness. Convinced that she had completely recovered from her illness, the governor felt that she ought to be freed and returned to her family, but first he had to consult with the Board of Punishments to see if it could be done. In his letter to the board, the governor made special note of the fact that many female prisoners, because they could not take advantage of the substatutes of 1801 and 1814, all too frequently languished and died in prison while awaiting an amnesty—their only chance to be freed. He asked the board to spare Wang this pitiful fate. The board, however, rejected the argument that she should be freed simply because she, like other female prisoners, could not take advantage of the substatutes of 1801 and 1814. The board pointed out that the most appropriate sentence for insane killers was life imprisonment, and that *liuyang chengsi* was only an extralegal benevolence. Moreover, the board was concerned that a dangerous precedent could be set if they freed Wang. The government would have to accommodate similar requests from male prisoners who were not sole surviving sons. To avoid undermining the principle of *liuyang chengsi* as well as the status quo, the board ruled against releasing Wang to the custody of her family (ibid., 3022–24).

It is clear from the cases discussed here that *liuyang chengsi* was a privilege to be dispensed at the emperor's grace and not an inalienable right. State sponsorship of filial piety did not mean that requests for commutation on the grounds of *liuyang chengsi* would be granted readily. In fact, in the eyes of the officials, the commission of a crime in itself branded the criminal an unfilial son. Thus it was with extreme skepticism that the government reviewed *liuyang chengsi* petitions. This attitude was not confined to the Qing, but, as an incident described by Tung-tsu Ch'ü shows, was one of very long standing:

> In 1173 the case of a man who had beaten another to death was reported to the emperor by the government. The criminal's parent was old and had no one to take care of him. Emperor [Shizong] (1161–1189) of the [Jin] dynasty said, "This man forgot his parents merely because he was angry. How can he have a mind to care for his parent? He should be sentenced according to the law" (Ch'ü 1961, 77)

Perhaps it was precisely because the government valued filial piety so highly that it was so stringent in its dispensation of *liuyang chengsi*.

There is no indication that the Board of Punishments employed a tougher set of criteria (other than the five-years-after-recovery rule) to evaluate petitions from criminals who ran afoul of the law because of their madness. It seems that as long as the officials were satisfied that a prisoner had fully recovered, his or her petition was given the same kind of deliberate scrutiny as those from ordinary prisoners.

We have seen in this chapter how the legal system wrestled with conflicting interests and values. Throughout the entire Qing period the government pushed hard to maintain the premier position occupied by the family in society; virtues such as filial piety, respect for the aged, and obedience toward superordinate relatives were promoted aggressively through a variety of ways and means. The legal system was one of the means employed to bolster the family and the message was clear: transgressions against the family and violations of the persons of superiors were regarded as serious offenses, not just social but criminal as well. The principle of aggravation, established long before the Qing dynasty, was continued and maintained by the Manchu state. On the other hand, from its earliest years, the Qing government had embraced the ancient doctrine that clemency must be shown to the inadvertent offender, regardless of the severity of the crime. Thus insane murderers were given special clemency; the only exceptions were those guilty of treason or parricide. It is clear from the intrafamily homicide laws presented in this chapter that the government was not willing to extend its hard line to include other forms of intrafamily violence. Another conflict was between the institution of *liuyang chengsi*, which allowed prisoners to return home to serve aged parents or to continue ancestral sacrifices, and the concern over public safety. In the end, the welfare of the public was considered more important and the government added more stringent conditions to the eligibility requirements for insane prisoners. Lawmakers were able to perform juridical acrobatics to obtain a reasonable resolution and to maintain an acceptable balance.

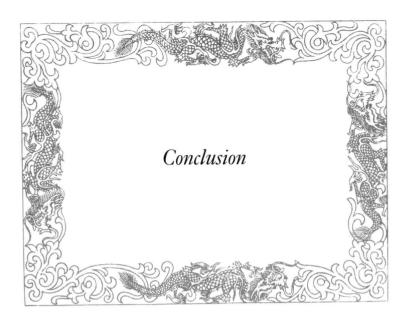

Conclusion

THE TRANSFORMATION OF MADNESS from illness to deviance in Qing China was a product of the drive on the part of the central government to control and regulate practically all aspects of life. This near-obsession was rooted in the history of the conquest of China by the alien Manchus and subsequent efforts at consolidation. The reestablishment of the *baojia* and *dibao* systems as police control agents contributed significantly to the formulation of a coherent policy toward the insane.

The first step toward the criminalization of madness was the decision to make mandatory the registration and confinement of all insane persons. This policy would have been inconceivable without the *baojia* and *dibao* systems. The Qing was unquestionably an autocratic state, but it was far from being totalitarian. In spite of numerous attempts on the part of the central government to extend its authority to all levels of society, effective state power stopped at the district (the lowest administrative) level. Beyond that, for any regulatory program to work, the government had to rely on the cooperation of the local gentry, village leaders, clan elders, and heads of households. The Qing had hoped to use the restored *baojia* system to extend its reach beyond the district level, but as Kung-chuan Hsiao has shown, a conspiracy of inaction, involving precisely those leaders whom the government had counted on for help, rendered the system impotent. The program to register and confine all the insane people and to make local authorities, neighbors, and family members accountable for their conduct failed to accomplish the goal for which it was originally intended, that is, to segregate a potentially dangerous (in the minds of high-ranking law-enforcement officials) segment of the population from the rest of society. Its failure is emblematic of the cultural resistance to the extension of state power in traditional China.

Since the violent nature of madness was well known to physicians long before the Qing, the government's determination that the insane constituted a potentially dangerous segment of society was not instigated by new medical knowledge. Indeed, the absence of any significant role played by physicians in the discussions on criminal insanity is telling. The official understanding of criminal insanity remained virtually unchanged throughout the Qing period. The debates that sometimes consumed jurists centered primarily around two issues. One was the struggle to reconcile the need to protect society with the long-held concept of justice. The other was the desire of some officials to serve the retributive purpose of punishment. Just as the Qing notion of criminal insanity cannot be traced to new medical discoveries, neither were subsequent legislative actions informed by any new understanding of madness.

In a sense, the response of the Qing state to the problem of madness was limited by Chinese culture and tradition. The lack of medical input in the discourse is a case in point. Physicians' remarkable lack of clout stemmed from a Confucian bias of long standing: devaluation of the worth (and therefore status) of specialists and professionals. Specialized knowledge, for example, was regarded as *xiaodao*, or "petty teachings," and in a key passage in the *Analects* of Confucius, the point is made that high-minded men do not occupy themselves with them. Paul Unschuld traced the stigmatization of medicine in China to Zhu Xi (1130–1200): "[Zhu Xi], the outstanding philosopher of neo-Confucianism, annotated the classic Confucian authors of antiquity, and in this context made a value judgment on medicine which remained effective for centuries" (1979, 38). What Zhu Xi did was to render "petty" specialized work such as medicine. Orthodox Confucianists, throughout the centuries, had taken practitioners of medicine to task for their pettiness and, by extension, moral turpitude. And because orthodox Confucianists dominated the political scene during the Qing period, there was little possibility that the learned opinions of physicians would be solicited. The intense rivalry between the schools of warmth-restorationists and heat purgers most likely further undermined the credibility of medical practitioners.

Even after the government moved to institutionalize its response to madness—that is, to register and confine the insane throughout the empire—no attempt was made to create special places of confinement for this new class of deviants. The new substatutes continued to specify the home as the primary (and preferred) incarceration site. Only when families could not meet the security requirements would local jails be used. The government seems to have believed that the family as a social unit was strong enough not only to continue its traditional function of caring for sick members, but also to accept the new responsibility of surveillance and control, for the good of the family as a whole. It was perhaps only natural that the Qing government would hold such a conviction; after all, it had invested considerable energy and resources in promoting and bolstering the Neo-Confucian model of the family. For example, as was noted in Chapter One, the biweekly village lectures and annual community drinking ceremonies, given new life and meaning by the Manchu conquerors early in the Qing period, were designed to drill traditional family values into the minds of the people. Perhaps the government succeeded too well in its effort to strengthen family ties. The mandatory registration-and-confinement program failed ultimately because people were unwilling to condemn their kin to a felon's existence. Additionally, the stigmatization of madness discouraged families from openly acknowledging the condition. Neighbors were unwilling to act as informants and enforcers because, as the old saying goes, "Each household sweeps only the snow gathered on its porch; who cares about the frost on others' roofs?" Thus, the response of Qing society to the problem of madness was shaped by culture and tradition.

A topic such as madness begs cross-cultural comparison, especially since its transformation from illness to a form of criminal deviance in China was so contrary to its European metamorphosis from deviance to illness. The English social historian Andrew T. Scull presents an excellent account of the English experience. In England, the push to segregate lunatics from able-bodied indigents was propelled by economic forces that were transforming society in the eighteenth and nineteenth centuries. Beginning in the eighteenth century, workhouses rapidly took the place of almshouses in the treatment of the poor. Founders of workhouses believed that old-style poor relief reinforced behavior that perpetuated impoverishment of the indigents, vagrants, and otherwise dislocated poor. Their solution was the establishment of institutions to house and put these people to work. Living conditions were made deliberately unattractive, so that "all save the truly needy and 'deserving' poor could be deterred from applying for relief" and those who did so would be motivated to acquire necessary skills and move out to become a part of the work force as soon as possible (1979, 22–35). By the late eighteenth century, as the capitalist system became more firmly entrenched and the need for a large pool of cheap laborers was more acutely felt, the move to separate disabled poor from the able-bodied in the workhouses was set apace. It was at this juncture and in this context that lunatics came under special attention:

A single mad or distracted person in the community produced problems of a wholly different sort from those the same person would have produced if placed with other deviants within the walls of an institution. The order and discipline of the whole workhouse were threatened by the presence of a madman who, even by threats and punishment, could neither be persuaded nor induced to conform to the regulations. And besides, by its very nature, the workhouse was ill-suited to provide a secure safe-keeping for those who might pose a threat to life or property. (Scull 1979, 40–41)

It was thus that the insane came to be identified as a distinct subset within the deviant population. The impetus for such a development came primarily from the demands of a capitalist economy and not, as in the case in Qing China, those of law and order. In England it was only fitting that the treatment of lunatics became a trade as private entrepreneurs recognized a new money-making opportunity.

The birth of madhouses generated new concerns, for the nineteenth century was also the Age of Reform in England. Many moral and social reformers, most of them Evangelicals and Benthamites, were disturbed by the coercive methods employed by proprietors of madhouses; they regarded the whip, the chain, the straitjacket, and the darkened room as cruel, degrading, and counterproductive. They proposed instead the use of moral suasion rather than physical coercion to refit the incarcerated lunatic for eventual reintegration into society. Their campaign for "moral treatment" of the insane gradually convinced the educated public that asylums could do more than merely segregate lunatics from society; they could also cure them (Walton 1981, 166). Madness came to be regarded as a condition that could be treated and cured by a regimen of moral education. The shift of emphasis from confinement to cure eventually pitted reformers (moral managers) against medical practitioners and ushered in the next phase in the social history of psychiatry in England. In the case of Qing China, such a confrontation did not materialize because, in the first instance, Confucian moralists, being members of the educated elite, did not subscribe to popular conceptions of madness that implicate moral turpitude in the myriad causes of the condition. Second, Confucian reformers, being generalists and not specialists, were concerned about larger and broader issues such as ethics of government or society as a whole, not issues as narrowly focused as the moral state of mind of lunatics. Third, Qing physicians did not—and, given the weight of tradition, could not—organize themselves into professional societies that carried political clout; thus, even if reformers had launched a campaign to cure madness with moral education and management, they would not have been in a position to advance a counterattack.

It was the political clout of medical societies that eventually won physicians monopoly over the treatment of the insane in England. Through persistent lobbying efforts directed at all levels of government, they persuaded officials as well as members of Parliament (especially those in the House of Lords) that insanity was a disease and that diagnosing the illness required expertise that only medical practitioners could provide. By the mid-nineteenth century, the law recognized only medical doctors as certifiers of insanity (Scull 1979, chap. 4; McCandless 1981, 341). [Note: In France, too, physicians were able to gain a similar monopoly. For a detailed account of this fascinating process, see Jan Goldstein's *Console and Classify: The French Psychiatric Profession in the Nineteenth Century* (1987).]

The transformation in China of madness from illness to criminal deviance did not mean that the Qing adopted a callous attitude toward the insane. To be sure, the mandatory registration-and-confinement program created hardship for both the afflicted and their families, yet Qing judicial authorities tried very hard to preserve the special place in traditional Chinese law occupied by the sick, a category that, since the Later Han period, had always included the insane. On balance, insane criminals fared much better than their sane counterparts. Even when they appeared disadvantaged by their affliction, as in the case of their limited eligibility for amnesties and pardons, their predicament was a product of the government's concern for public safety, and not prejudice against madness itself.

The saga of Qing legislative response to the problem of criminal insanity reveals a system that was remarkably flexible, so that it was able to deal rather quickly not only with social change—such as growing unrest in Sichuan due to vagrancy and tenant unrest or the threat of sectarian uprisings—but also with deficiencies in the laws themselves. Since many of the new laws and procedures were responses to initiatives taken by individual officials, they point to the fact that initiatives did matter in the Qing bureaucracy, that they were not routinely consumed by the organization, never to be seen again. The legislative history also adds to our understanding of the process called "Confucianization of law." The single-homicide laws provide a good example of this: Qing jurists were engaged in a ceaseless effort to rectify what they perceived to be imperfections in the laws, not only to deter tendencies toward deviancy (a Legalist impulse) but also to ensure fair and humane treatment of the criminally insane (a Confucian concern). The humane quality of the Qing laws discussed in this study is truly remarkable, especially in light of the fact that criminals in China did not have lawyers such as John Erskine or Alexander Cockburn to formulate arguments in their defense. It is equally noteworthy that, even without the advocacy system, Qing jurists were able to arrive at tests of insanity that were similar to those delineated in the landmark M'Naghten Case of 1843.

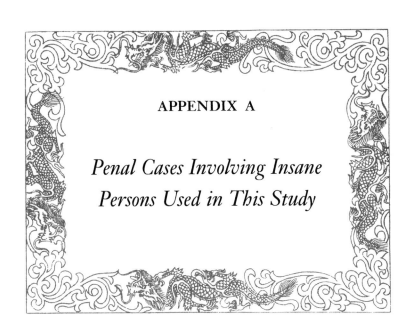

APPENDIX A

Penal Cases Involving Insane Persons Used in This Study

Chronological List of Penal Cases Involving Insane Persons Used in This Study

Date	Status	Sex	Offense	Victim	Penalty/Comments	Sources
1. 1697	Commoner	F	Homicide	Husband	None	*Li'an chuanji*, 22: 26a–26b.
2. 1703	Commoner	F	Homicide	Mother-in-law	Decapitation after assizes	*Cheng'an zhiyi*, 19: 39a–39b.
3. 1731	Commoner	M	Multiple homicide	4 of another family	12.42 taels of silver 4 times	Ibid., 42a–42b.
4. 1732	Commoner	M	Homicide	Wife	Confinement at home	Ibid., 41a–41b.
5. 1735	Commoner	M	Homicide	No relation	12.42 taels	Ibid., 43a–43b.
6. 1753	Commoner	M	Multiple homicide	4 of another family	12.42 taels, 4 times	Xue Yunsheng, *Duli cunyi*, 682–83.
7. 1756	Commoner	M	Homicide	Brother	Decapitation after assizes	*Cheng'an xinpian*, 9:21a–22b.
8. 1758	Commoner	M	Robbery/ homicide	Stranger	12.42 taels, imprisonment	Ibid., 14a–19a.
9. 1759	Commoner	M	Homicide	Younger *dagong* cousin	Strangulation after assizes	Ibid., 20a–20b.
10. 1760	Commoner	M	Homicide	Mother's stepson's wife	Strangulation after assizes	Ibid., 12a–13b.
11. 1766	Commoner	M	Multiple homicide	4 of another family	12.42 taels, 4 times	*Dingli huipian*, 13:73a–76b.
12. 1786	Commoner	M	Treason		*Lingchi*	*Qianlong shilu*, 14397–98, 14415, 14459.
13. 1786	Commoner	M	Homicide	*Sima* elder	Decapitation after assizes	*Boan xinpian*, 1783–89.

No.	Year	Status	Sex	Crime	Victim/Relation	Punishment	Source
14.	1789	Commoner	M	Multiple homicide	5 unrelated persons	Strangulation after assizes (governor's request for immediate decapitation denied)	Ibid., 1783.
15.	1789	Commoner	M	Multiple homicide	Killed sister-in-law, nephew, neighbor; wounded father	Immediate decapitation	*Daqing lüli buiji bilan*, 3736–37.
16.	1792	Commoner	M	Homicide	Mother-in-law	Decapitation after assizes	*Xing'an huilan*, 2120.
17.	1805	Commoner	M	Homicide	*Sima* elder	Decapitation after assizes	*Jiaqing shilu*, 2179.
18.	1805	Commoner	M	Homicide	No relation	Strangulation after assizes	Ibid.
19.	1805	Commoner	M	Homicide	No relation	Strangulation after assizes	Ibid.
20.	1805	Commoner	M	Homicide	No relation	Strangulation after assizes	Ibid.
21.	1806	Commoner	M	Stealing head of executed criminal		Exile	Ibid., 2370.
22.	1806	Commoner	M	Homicide	Female junior relative	Life term	*Xing'an huilan*, 2113–15.
23.	1806	Commoner	M	Homicide	Daughter-in-law	Life term	Ibid.
24.	1806	Commoner	M	False accusation		Confinement at home	Ibid., 2128.
25.	1806	Bannerman	M	False accusation		Sent back to banner for confinement at home	Ibid.

Appendix A (*continued*)

Date	Status	Sex	Offense	Victim	Penalty/Comments	Sources
26. 1806	Commoner	F	Homicide	Husband	Decapitation after assizes	*Jiaqing shilu*, 2415–16, 2424–25.
27. 1808	Commoner	F	Homicide	*Sima* elder	Decapitation after assizes	*Xing'an huilan*, 2124.
28. 1809	Commoner	M	Multiple homicide	3 kinsmen	Immediate decapitation	Ibid., 2125.
29. 1809	Commoner	M	Multiple homicide	Wife, son	Strangulation after assizes	*Shuotie leipian*, 2:18a–19a.
30. 1810	Commoner	M	Homicide	Wife	Life imprisonment (released in 1819; *liuyang chengsi*)	*Xing'an huilan*, 2119; *Shuotie leipian*, 2:41a–42b.
31. 1811	Commoner	M	Registration and confinement			*Lüliguan shuotie*, no pagination.
32. 1811	Commoner	M	Multiple homicide	Neighbor, neighbor's wife	Strangulation after assizes	*Xing'an huilan*, 2112–13.
33. 1812	Commoner	F	Homicide	Husband	Immediate decapitation	Ibid., 2123.
34. 1812	Commoner	M	Homicide	Stepfather	Decapitation after assizes	Ibid., 2124.
35. 1813	Commoner	M	Homicide	Daughter	Life term	Ibid., 2116–17.
36. 1813	Commoner	M	Homicide	Wife	Life term	Ibid., 2120.
37. 1813	Commoner	M	Homicide	Younger brother	Failed to recover; life term	Ibid., 2119–2120.

No. Year	Status	Sex	Crime	Relation	Punishment	Source
38. 1813	Commoner	M	Breaking and entering		Killed while committing crime	*XBJC*, 11:2a–2b.
39. 1814	Commoner	M	Multiple homicide	Sister-in-law; niece	Strangulation after assizes	*Lüliguan shuotie*, no pagination.
40. 1816	Commoner	M	Assault	Aunt	Strangulation after assizes	*Xing'an huilan*, 2121.
41. 1816	Indentured servant	M	Multiple homicide	Master, one other person	Immediate decapitation	*XBJC*, 19:32b–33a.
42. 1817	Commoner	M	Multiple homicide	Parents, wife, sister-in-law	*Lingchi* with extra slices plus exposure of head	*Yuedong cheng'an chupian*, 13:24b–25a.
43. 1817	Commoner	M	Homicide	No relation	Strangulation after assizes	*XBJC*, 23:2a–2b.
44. 1817	Commoner	M	Assault	No relation	80 strokes, 2-year jail term, 5.32 taels	Ibid., 21:6a–6b.
45. 1818	Commoner	M	Multiple homicide	Wife, uncle	Immediate decapitation	*Xing'an huilan*, 2122.
46. 1818	Commoner	M	Homicide	Neighbor	Life term	Ibid., 2118.
47. 1821	Commoner	M	False accusation	No relation	Life term	*XBJC*, 23:2a–2b.
48. 1822	Commoner	M	Homicide	Father	Killed by mother, corpse ordered mutilated in public *lingchi*	Ibid., 21:6a–6b.
49. 1823	Commoner	M	Homicide	Father	*Lingchi*	*Xing'an huilan*, 2763–64.
50. 1824	Commoner	M	Homicide	Uncle's creditor	Died in prison while serving life term	*Yuedong cheng'an*, 13:28b.
51. 1824	Commoner	M	Homicide	4 persons	Decapitation after assizes	*Xing'an huilan*, 2125–26.

Appendix A (*continued*)

Date	Status	Sex	Offense	Victim	Penalty/Comments	Sources
52. 1825	Commoner	M	Assault	No relation	Military exile 5 years after recovery	Ibid., 2126.
53. 1825	Commoner	M	Homicide	*Xiaogong* elder	Immediate decapitation	*Xing'an huilan xupian*, 273–75.
54. 1826	Commoner	M	Homicide	No relation	Life term	*Xuean chumu xupian, Fengbing sharen,* 14a–14b.
55. 1826	Commoner	M	Assault	*Dagong* cousin	100 blows, 2,000 *li* exile	*Xing'an huilan,* 2121.
56. 1826	Commoner	M	Commandeered a donkey, rode it "wildly," down a public street		Put in prison because his family did not have barred room at home	Ibid., 2113.
57. 1827	Commoner	M	Assault	Uncle	Strangulation after assizes	Ibid., 2121–22.
58. 1828	Commoner	M	Homicide	*Sima* elder	Decapitation after assizes	Ibid., 2127.
59. 1830	Commoner	M	Assault	Banner captain	12.42 taels, imprisonment	Ibid., 2124–25.
60. 1831	Commoner	F	Homicide	Daughter-in-law	100 blows, 3 years exile. Penalty redeemed with money, confinement at home	Ibid., 2124.

No. Year	Status	Sex	Crime	Relation	Sentence	Source
61. 1832	Deputy magistrate	M	Forging seal of another official		Dismissed from civil service, life imprisonment at native place	Ibid., 2126–27.
62. 1833	Commoner	M	False accusation	Former employee	Life term	Ibid., 4515.
63. 1840	Commoner	M	Homicide		Life term	Xing'an huilan xupian, 3022–24.
64. 1841	Commoner	M	Homicide	No relation	Strangulation after assizes	Ibid., 3036–37.
65. 1841	Commoner	M	Homicide	No relation	Strangulation after assizes, released in 1849	Ibid., 317–18.
66. 1843	Commoner	M	Homicide	Son	Short-term imprisonment, eligible for release 5 years after recovery	Ibid., 2995–96.
67. 1843	Commoner	M	Homicide	Natural father's adoptive mother	Unknown	Ibid., 3965–68.
68. 1845	Commoner	M	Registration and confinement; committed to prison by elder brother			Ibid., 2993–95.
69. 1846	Commoner	M	Homicide	Brother's child-bride	Life term, released 1846	Lixue xinpian, 10:3b–4a.
70. 1848	Commoner	M	Homicide	No relation	Strangulation after assizes	Xing'an huilan xupian, 3033–36.

Appendix A (continued)

Date	Status	Sex	Offense	Victim	Penalty/Comments	Sources
71. 1849	Commoner	F	Homicide	Stepson	Crime committed earlier, set free in 1849 because of failing eyesight	Ibid., 2995–96.
72. 1852	Commoner	M	Assault	Elder brother	Imprisonment, set free in 1852	Ibid., 3737.
73. 1853	Commoner	M	Homicide	Stepson	Imprisonment, eligible for release after 5 years	Ibid., 2997–98.
74. 1853	Commoner	M	Homicide	Daoist priest/landlord	Sent back for retrial	Ibid., 3024–27.
75. 1854	Commoner	M	Homicide	No relation	Sent back for retrial	Ibid., 3027–29.
76. 1854	Commoner	M	Assault	Xiaogong elder	Board of Punishments rejected 1854 request for release	Ibid., 3038–39.
77. 1857	Commoner	M	Multiple homicide	Wife, sister-in-law	Strangulation after assizes	Qiushen bijiao huian, 2:16b.
78. 1858	Commoner	F	Homicide	Husband	Immediate decapitation, later reduced by emperor to decapitation after assizes	Xing'an huilan xupian, 3042–43.
79. 1858	Commoner	M	Homicide	Dagong cousin	Immediate decapitation, reduced to decapitation after assizes, further reduced to life imprisonment	Ibid., 3039–42.

No. Year	Status	Sex	Crime	Victim	Sentence	Source
80. 1859	Commoner	M	Homicide		Life term	Ibid, 2998–3002.
81. 1860	Sergeant	M	Homicide		Imprisonment	Xing'an huilan, 5008.
82. 1867	Commoner	M	Homicide	Wife	Life sentence but could be released 5 years after recovery to serve parents	Quisben bijiao buian, 2:16b.
83. 1867	Commoner	M	Homicide	Ex-employer's wife	Retrial	Xing'an huilan xu-pian, 3003–5.
84. 1868	Commoner	M	Multiple homicide	2 unrelated persons	Strangulation after assizes	Quisben bijiao buian, 2:16b.
85. 1868	Bannerman	M	Gang rape	Bannerwoman	Re-investigation ordered	Xing'an huilan xu-pian, 4437.
86. 1868	Prisoner	M	Homicide	Cell mate	Trial deferred 2 to 3 years pending recovery	Ibid., 3005–3007.
87. 1870	Commoner	M	Multiple homicide	Wife's relatives	Unknown	Quisben bijiao buian, 2:16b.
88. 1870	Commoner	M	Homicide	Wife	Strangulation after assizes	Xing'an huilan xu-pian, 3007–12.
89. 1870	Commoner	M	Multiple homicide	2 unrelated persons	Strangulation after assizes	Quisben bijiao buian, 2:16b.
90. 1870	Commoner (barber)	M	Multiple homicide	Magistrate, 2 others	Lingchi, exposure of head	Xing'an huilan xu-pian, 2351–55.
91. 1870	Bannerman	M	Multiple homicide	2 persons	Strangulation after assizes	Ibid., 3019–22.
92. 1871	Commoner	M	Homicide	No relation	Strangulation after assizes	Quisben bijiao buian, 2:16b.

Appendix A (continued)

Date	Status	Sex	Offense	Victim	Penalty/Comments	Sources
93. 1875	Commoner	M	Homicide	Nephew	Temporary imprisonment, to be exiled 5 years after recovery	*Lixue xinpian*, 10:4b.
94. 1875	Commoner	M	Multiple homicide	Uncle, aunt, cousin	Immediate decapitation	Ibid., 5a.
95. 1875	Commoner	M	Abduction	Woman	Kept in jail as material witness	*Jiansha ousbang chuan'an shili gao*, "Huguang si: Wu Zhaisheng," no pagination.
96. 1875	Commoner	M	Assault	2 persons	100 blows, 3 years in exile, reduced to imprisonment	*Lixue xinpian*, 10:2a.
97. 1880	Prisoner	M	Homicide	Cell mate	Unknown	Ibid., 5a–5b.
98. 1880	Commoner	M	Barging into palace grounds; tirade against government		Strangulation after assizes	*Xing'an huilan*, 4893.
99. 1880	Uncle of eunuch	M	Entering palace grounds without permission		100 blows	Ibid.
100. 1881	Assistant magistrate	M	Writing abusive letters to superiors		100 blows	Ibid., 5061.

101. 1881	Commoner	M	Multiple homicide	Aunt, wife, son	Immediate decapitation with petition for reduction to decapitation after assizes	*Lixue xinpian,* 10:2a–2b.
102. 1882	Commoner	M	Multiple homicide	2 kinsmen	Military exile to remote region after recovery	Ibid., 2b.
103. 1885	Commoner	M	Homicide	Adoptive mother	*lingchi*	*Xing'an huilan,* 4976.
104. 1891	Commoner	M	Multiple homicide	Wife, son, daughter	Life term	*Lixue xinpian,* 10:2b–3a.
105. 1892	Commoner	M	Homicide	Jailer	Life term	Ibid., 3b–4a.

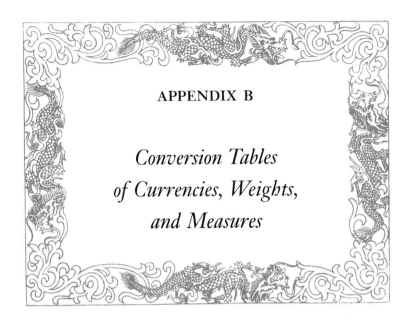

APPENDIX B

*Conversion Tables
of Currencies, Weights,
and Measures*

Currencies
1 *tael*　= 1 Chinese ounce, or 1.208 English ounces, of pure silver

Weights
1 picul (*shi*　) = 100 catties (*jin*　) = 133⅓ pounds
1 catty = 16 taels = 60.453 kilograms
1 tael = 1⅓ ounces = 37.783 grams
16.8 piculs = 1 long ton
16.54 piculs = 1 metric ton
1 peck (*don*　) = 316 cubic inches

Measures
1 *li*　= ⅓ mile = ½ kilometer
1 *chi*　= 1 Chinese foot or cubit = 14.1 inches

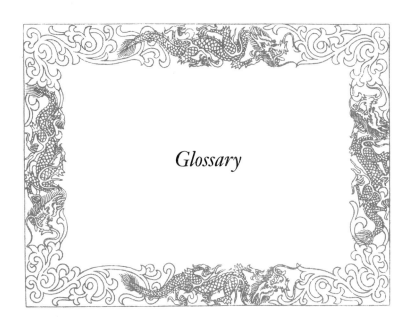

Glossary

ai 呆
bao 保
baojia 保甲
changli zhiwai 常理之外
Chen Shiduo 陳士鐸
chunyu 蠢愚
dagong 大功
Danqi xinfa 丹溪心法
dian 癲
diankuang 癲狂
dibao 地保
dousha 鬪殺
fa 法
feng 瘋
fengfa wuzhi 瘋發無知

gongqing wangming 恭請王命
guoshisha 過失殺
gusha 故殺
Hejian liushu 河間六書
Hua Tuo 華陀
huadian 花癲
Huangdi neijing (lingshu; suwen) 黃帝內經(靈樞;素問)
jia 甲
Jingyue chuanshu 景岳全書
jiuqing 九卿
kaocheng 考成
kuang 狂
Kunzhi yuannian 坤治元年
li (propriety) 禮
li (substatute) 例
lingchi 淩遲
Liu Wansu 劉元素
Liu Wenshu 劉溫舒
liuyang chengsi 留養承祀
lü 律
mousha 謀殺
Nanjing 難經
pai 牌
pingchang 平常
ping su ji wu ling fan 平素既無淩犯
qi 氣
Qianjin yaofang 千金要方
Qianjin yifang 千金翼方
qigong 期功
qingshi 情實
qingzhi 情志
renming 人命
ruxue 儒學
sangang 三綱
sanshe 三赦
sha 殺
Shanghan lun 傷寒論
shi'e 十惡
Shishi bilu 石室秘錄
sima 緦麻
Sun Simiao 孫思邈
tongzong 同宗
Wang Mengying 王孟英
Weisheng baojian 衛生寶鑑
wenbu pai 溫補派

Wu Jutong 吳鞠通
wufu 五服
wusha 誤殺
wuxing 五行
wuyun liuqi 五運六氣
wuzhi 無知
xianghuo 相火
xiangyue 鄉約
xiaodao 小道
xiaogong 小功
xinbing 心病
xisha 戲殺
yangjing 陽經
yinjing 陰經
yin feng sha ren 因瘋殺人
ze 責
zhancui 斬衰
zuzhang 族長
zuzheng 族正
Zhang Conzheng 張從政
Zhang Ji 張機
Zhang Jiebin 張介賓
Zhongzang jing 中藏經
Zhu Zhenheng 朱震亨
zicui 齊衰
zuoling 佐領

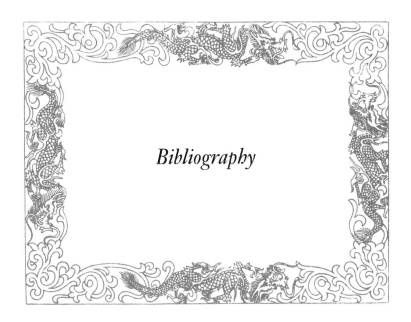

Bibliography

Abbreviations

BXD   *Biji xiaoshuo daguan*
DXXA   *Daqing xianxing xinglü anyü*
YBCL   *Yibu chuanlu (Qinding gujin tushu jicheng yibu chuanlu)*
XBJC   *Xingbu bizhao jiajian cheng'an*

Original Sources

Biji xiaoshuo daguan 筆記小說大觀. 1974. 3d, 4th, and 5th series. Taipei.
Boan huipian 駁案彙編. 1886. Zhu Meishen 朱梅臣, comp.
Boan xinpian 駁案新編. 1968 Quan Shichao 全士潮, comp. Reprint, Taipei.
Cheng'an xinpian 成案新編. 1763. Wen Wobi 閔我備, comp.

Cheng'an zhiyi 成案質疑. 1755. Hong Hongxu 洪弘緒 and Rao Han 饒瀚, comps.

Daqing huidian 大清會典. 1963. Reprint, Taipei: Qiwen Book Co.

Daqing huidian shili 大清會典事例. 1963. Reprint, Taipei: Qiwen Publishing Co.

Daqing lichao shilu 大清歷朝實錄. 1964. Reprint, Taipei: Huawen Book Co.

Daqing lüli huiji bianlan 大清律例彙輯便覽. 1975. Reprint, Taipei: Wen Hai Publishing Co.

Daqing xianxing xinglü anyü 大清現行刑律按語. 1908. Shen Jiaben 沈家本, comp.

Dingli huipian 定例彙編. 1762–1883. Jiangxi Judicial Commissioner's Office, comp.

Jiansha oushang chuan'an shili gao 姦殺毆傷全案事例稿. Guangxu period. edition.

Jiaqing shilu 嘉慶實錄. See *Daqing lichao shilu.*

Li'an chuanji 例案全集. 1722. Zhang Guangyue 張光月, comp.

Lixue xinpian 例學新編. 1907. Yang Shixiang 楊士驤, comp.

Lüliguan shuotie 律例館說帖. 1805–1814. Statutes Commission, comp.

Pu Songling 蒲松齡. 1976. *Liaozhai zhiyi* 聊齋志異. Shanghai: Commercial Press.

Qianlong shilu 乾隆實錄. See *Daqing lichao shilu.*

Qinding gujin tushu jicheng 欽定古今圖書集成. 1884. Chen Menglei 陳夢雷, comp.

Qinding gujin tushu jicheng yibu chuanlu 欽定古今圖書集成醫部全錄. 1962. Reprint, Beijing: Renmin weisheng Publishing Co.

Qiushen bijiao huian 秋審比較彙案. See *Boan huipian.*

Shen Jiaben 沈家本. 1964. *Shen Jiyi xiansheng yishu jiapian* 沈寄簃先生遺書甲編. Reprint, Taipei: Wen Hai Publishing Co.

Shizu shilu (Shizu zhang huangdi shilu) 世祖章皇帝實錄. 1937. Tokyo: Ōkura Publishing Co.

Shuotie leipian 說帖類編. 1836. Statutes Commission, comp.

Tushu jicheng 圖書集成. See *Qinding gujin tushu jicheng yibu chuantu.*

Wang Shihong 王士雄. 1957. *Wangshi yian yizhu* 王氏醫案繹注. Shanghai.

Xing'an huilan 刑案匯覽. 1968. Reprint, Taipei: Wen Hai Publishing Co.

Xing'an huilan xupian 刑案匯覽續編. 1970. Reprint, Taipei: Wen Hai Publishing Co.

Xingbu bizhao jiajian cheng'an 刑部比照加減成案. 1834. Xu Lian 許槤 and Xiong Wo 熊莪, comps.

Xue Yunsheng 薛允升. 1970. *Duli cunyi* 讀例存疑. Reprint, Taipei: Chinese Materials and Research Aids Service Center.

Xuean chumu xupian 學案初模續編. 1881. Yi Libu 伊里布, comp.

Yuedong cheng'an chupian 粵東成案初編, 1882. Zhu Shu 朱樞 comp.

Zengding tongxing tiaoli 增訂通行條例. 1883. Guo Ying 國英, comp.

Chinese and Japanese Secondary Works

Chen Guyuan 陳顧遠. 1934. *Zongguo fazhi shi* 中國法制史. Shanghai: Commercial Press.

Jia Dedao 賈得道. 1979. *Zhongguo yixue shilüe* 中国医学史略. Taiyuan: Shanxi People's Press.

Maeno Naoaki 前野直彬. 1975. *Chūgoku shosetsu shi ko* 中国小説史考. Tokyo: Akiyama Shoten.

Nakamura Shigeo 中村茂夫. 1973. *Shindai keihō kenkyū* 清代刑法研究. Tokyo: University of Tokyo Press.

Niida Noboru 仁井田陞. 1952. *Chūgoku hōseishi* 中國法制史. Tokyo: Iwanami Shoten.

Nishida Taichirō 西田太一郎. 1974. *Chūgoku keihōshi kenkyū* 中国刑法史研究. Tokyo: Iwanami Shoten.

Qin Bowei 秦伯未. 1959. *Qingdai mingyi yian jinghua* 清代名医医案精华. Shanghai: Science and Technology Press.

Suzuki Chūsei 鈴木中正. 1974. *Chūgoku ni okeru kakumei tō shūkyō* 中国史における革命と宗教. Tokyo: University of Tokyo Press.

Yang Honglie 楊鴻烈. 1970. *Zhongguo falü fada shi* 中國法律發達史. Shanghai: Commercial Press.

Yazawa Toshihiko 矢沢利彦, comp. and trans. 1970. *lezusukai Chūgoku shokanshu* イエズス会中国書簡集. Vol. 1. Tokyo: Heibonsha.

Zhao Qinshi 趙琴仟. 1936. *Shenxian biji jinghua* 神仙筆記菁華. Shanghai.

Western Secondary Works

Alabaster, Ernest. 1968. *Notes and Commentaries on Chinese Criminal Law and Cognate Topics, with Special Relation to Ruling Cases.* Reprint, Taipei: Ch'eng-Wen Publishing Co.

Ahern, Emily. 1973. *The Cult of the Dead in a Chinese Village.* Stanford: Stanford University Press.

———. 1978. "Chinese-style and Western-style Doctors in Northern Taiwan." In *Culture and Healing in Asian Societies: Anthropological, Psychiatric, and Public Health Studies*, edited by Arthur Kleinman.

Baker, Hugh, D. R. 1974. *Chinese Family and Kinship.* New York: Columbia University Press.

Bodde, Derk. 1969. "Prison Life in Eighteenth-Century Peking." *Journal of the American Oriental Society* 89, no. 2: 311–333.

———. 1980. "Age, Youth, and Infirmity in the Law of Ch'ing China." In *Essays on China's Legal Tradition*, edited by Jerome Cohen, R. Randle Edwards, and Fu-mei Chang Chen.

Bodde, Derk, and Clarence Morris. 1973. *Law in Imperial China, Exemplified by 190 Ch'ing Dynasty Cases (Translated from the Hsing-an Huilan), with Historical, Social, and Juridical Commentaries.* Philadelphia: University of Pennsylvania Press.

Boswell, John, 1980. *Christianity, Social Tolerence and Homosexuality.* Chicago: University of Chicago Press.

Boulais, Gui. 1966. *Manuel du code Chinois.* Taipei: Ch'eng-Wen Publishing Co.

Bünger, Karl. 1950. "The Punishment of Lunatics and Negligents According to Classical Chinese Law." *Studia Serica* 9, no. 2:1–16.

Carroll, John, 1977. *Puritans, Paranoid, Remissive: A Sociology of Modern Culture.* London: Routledge and Kegan Paul.

Chan, Wing-tsit. 1973. *A Source Book in Chinese Philosophy.* Princeton: Princeton University Press.

Chen, Chang Fu-mei. 1970. "On Analogy in Ch'ing Law." *Harvard Journal of Asiatic Studies* 30:212–224.

———. 1975. "Local Control of Convicted Thieves in Eighteenth-Century China." In *Conflict and Control in Late Imperial China,* edited by Frederic Wakeman, Jr., and Carol Grant. Berkeley: University of California Press.

Chiu, Martha Li. 1981. "Insanity in Imperial China: A Legal Case Study." In *Normal and Abnormal Behavior in Chinese Culture,* edited by Arthur Kleinman and Tsung-yi Lin. Dordrecht, Holland: D. Reidel Publishing Co.

Ch'ü, T'ung-tsu. 1961. *Law and Society in Imperial China.* Paris: Mouton and Co.

———. 1969. *Local Government in China Under the Ch'ing.* Stanford: Stanford University Press.

Cohen, Jerome A., R. Randle Edwards, and Fu-mei Chang Chen, eds. 1980. *Essays on China's Legal Tradition.* Princeton: Princeton University Press.

Connor, Walter D. 1972. "The Manufacture of Deviance: The Case of the Soviet Purge, 1936–1938." *American Sociological Review* 32:403–13.

Conrad, Peter, and Joseph W. Schneider. 1980. *Deviance and Medicalization: From Badness to Sickness.* St. Louis: C. V. Mosby Co.

De Bary, Wm. Theodore. 1970. *Self and Society in Ming Thought.* New York: Columbia University Press.

Dennerline, Jerry. 1981. *The Chia-ting Loyalists: Confucian Leadership and Social Change.* New Haven: Yale University Press.

Digby, Anne. 1985. *Madness, Morality and Medicine: A Study of the York Retreat, 1796–1914.* Cambridge, England: Cambridge University Press.

Doré, Henry. 1966. *Researches Into Chinese Superstitions.* Reprint, Taipei: Ch'eng-Wen Publishing Co.

Eastman, Lloyd. 1988. *Family, Fields, and Ancestors: Constancy and Change in China's Social and Economic History, 1550–1949.* New York: Oxford University Press.

Eberhard, Wolfram. 1967. *Guilt and Sin in Traditional China.* Berkeley: University of California Press.

Eikemeier, Dieter, and Herbert Franke, eds. 1981. *State and Law in East Asia: Festschrift Karl Bünger*. Wiesbaden: Otto Harrassowitz.

Entenmann, Robert. 1980. "Sichuan and Qing Migration Policy." *Ch'ing-shih wen-t'i* 4, no. 4:35–54.

Erikson, Kai T. 1966. *Wayward Puritans: A Study in the Sociology of Deviance*. New York: Wiley.

Foucault, Michel. 1965. *Madness and Civilization: A History of Insanity in the Age of Reason*. New York: Plume Books.

———. 1979. *Discipline and Punish: The Birth of the Prison*. New York: Peregrin Books.

Gibbs, Jack P. 1981. *Norms, Deviance, and Social Control: Conceptual Matters*. New York: Elsevier.

Goldstein, Jan. 1987. *Console and Classify: The French Psychiatric Profession in the Nineteenth Century*. Cambridge, England: Cambridge University Press.

Goodrich, L. Carrington. 1966. *The Literary Inquisition of Ch'ien-Lung*. New York: Paragon Book Reprint Corp.

Gray, John Henry. 1878. *China: A History of the Laws, Manners, and Customs of the People*. 2 vols. London: Macmillan and Co.

Guy, R. Kent. 1987. *The Emperor's Four Treasuries: Scholars and the State in the Late Ch'ien-lung Era*. Cambridge, Mass.: Council on East Asian Studies, Harvard University.

Hegel, Robert E. 1981. *The Novel in Seventeenth Century* China. New York: Columbia University Press.

Hsiao, Kung-chuan. 1960. *Rural China: Imperial Control in the Nineteenth Century*. Seattle: University of Washington Press.

Hsü, Immanuel C. Y. 1970. *The Rise of Modern China*. New York: Oxford University Press.

Huang, Pei. 1974. *Autocracy at Work: A Study of the Yung-Cheng Period, 1723–35*. Bloomington: Indiana University Press.

Huang, Ray. 1981. *1587, A Year of No Significance: The Ming Dynasty In Decline*. New Haven: Yale University Press.

Hulsewé, A. F. P. 1955. *Remnants of Han Law*. Vol. 1. Leiden: E. J. Brill.

Jen, Yu-wen. 1970. "Ch'en Hsien-chang's Philosophy of the Natural." In *Self and Society in Ming Thought*, edited by Wm. Theodore de Bary.

Johnson, David. 1985. "Communication, Class, and Consciousness in Late Imperial China." In *Popular Culture in Late Imperial China*, edited by David Johnson, Andrew J. Nathan, and Evelyn S. Rawski.

Johnson, David, Andrew J. Nathan, and Evelyn S. Rawski, eds. 1985. *Popular Culture in Late Imperial China*. Berkeley: University of California Press.

Johnson, Wallace. 1979. *The T'ang Code*. Vol. 1, *General Principles*. Princeton: Princeton University Press.

Kahn, Harold. 1971. *Monarchy in the Emperor's Eyes: Image and Reality in the Ch'ien-lung Reign*. Cambridge, Mass.: Harvard University Press.

Kessler, Lawrence D. 1976. *K'ang-hsi and the Consolidation of Ch'ing Rule, 1661–1684*. Chicago: University of Chicago Press.

Kleinman, Arthur, ed. 1978. *Culture and Healing in Asian Societies: Anthropological, Psychiatric, and Public Health Studies*. Boston: G. K. Hall.

Kleinman, Arthur, and Tsung-yi Lin, eds. 1981. *Normal and Abnormal Behavior in Chinese Culture*. Dordrecht, Holland: D. Reidel Publishing Co.

Kuhn, Philip A. 1970. *Rebellion and Its Enemies in Late Imperial China: Militarization and Social Structure, 1796–1864*. Cambridge, Mass.: Harvard University Press.

Lamson, Robert D. 1935. *Social Pathology in China: A Source Book from the Study of Problems of Livelihood, Health, and the Family*. Shanghai: Commercial Press.

Langlois, John D., Jr. 1981. "Authority in Family Legislation." In *State and Law in East Asia: Festschrift Karl Bünger*, edited by Dieter Eikmeier and Herbert Franke.

Lin, Keh-Ming. 1981. "Traditional Chinese Medical Beliefs and Their Relevance for Mental Illness and Psychiatry." In *Normal and Abnormal Behavior in Chinese Culture*, edited by Arthur Kleinman and Tsung-yi Lin.

Lock, Margaret M. 1980. *East Asian Medicine in Urban Japan*. Berkeley: University of California Press.

McCandless, Peter. 1981. "Liberty and Lunacy: The Victorians and Wrongful Confinement." In *Madhouses, Mad-doctors, and Madmen: The Social History of Pyschiatry in the Victorian Era*, edited by Andrew Scull.

McKnight, Brian E. 1981. *The Quality of Mercy: Amnesties and Traditional Chinese Justice*. Honolulu: University Press of Hawaii.

Mair, Victor. 1985. "Language and Ideology in the *Sacred Edict*." In *Popular Culture in Late Imperial China*, edited by David Johnson, Andrew J. Nathan, and Evelyn S. Rawski.

Metzger, Thomas. 1973. *The Internal Organization of the Ch'ing Bureaucracy: Legal, Normative and Communication Aspects*. Cambridge, Mass.: Harvard University Press.

Naquin, Susan. 1976. *Millenarian Rebellion in China: The Eight Trigrams Uprising of 1813*. New Haven: Yale University Press.

————. 1981. *Shantung Rebellion: The Wang Lun Uprising of 1774*. New Haven: Yale University Press.

Naquin, Susan, and Evelyn S. Rawski. 1987. *Chinese Society in the Eighteenth Century*. New Haven: Yale University Press.

Needham, Joseph. 1956. *Science and Civilization in China*. Vol. 1. Cambridge, England: Cambridge University Press.

————. 1970. *Clerks and Craftsmen in China and the West*. Cambridge, England: Cambridge University Press.

—— and Lu Gwei-djen. 1980. *Celestial Lancets: A History and Rationale of Acupuncture and Moxa.* Cambridge, England: Cambridge University Press.

Ng, Vivien W. 1980. "Ch'ing Laws Concerning the Insane: An Historical Survey." *Ch'ing-shih wen-t'i* 4, no. 4:55–89.

——. 1987. "Ideology and Sexuality: Rape Laws in Qing China." *Journal of Asian Studies* 46, no. 1:57–70

Nye, Robert A. 1984. *Crime, Madness, and Politics in Modern France: The Medical Concept of National Decline.* Princeton: Princeton University Press.

Oxnam, Robert B. 1975. *Ruling from Horseback: Manchu Politics in the Oboi Regency 1661–1669.* Chicago: University of Chicago Press.

Parsons, James B. 1970. *The Peasant Rebellions of Late Ming Dynasty.* Tucson: University of Arizona Press.

Porkert, Manfred. 1974. *The Theoretical Foundation of Chinese Medicine: Systems of Correspondence.* Cambridge, Mass.: MIT Press.

Ropp, Paul. 1981. *Dissent in Early Modern China: Ju-lin wai-shih and Ch'ing Social Criticism.* Ann Arbor: University of Michigan Press.

Rosen, George. 1968. *Madness in Society.* New York: Harper & Row.

Rothman, David. 1971. *The Discovery of the Asylum: Social Order and Disorder in the New Republic.* Boston: Little, Brown and Co.

Rowe, William T. 1977. "A Note on Ti-Pao." *Ch'ing-shih wen-t'i* 3, no. 8:79–85.

Scull, Andrew T. 1979. *Museums of Madness: The Social Organization of Insanity in Nineteenth-Century England.* London: Allen Lane.

——. ed. 1981a. *Madhouses, Mad-doctors, and Madmen: The Social History of Psychiatry in the Victorian Era.* Philadelphia: University of Philadelphia Press.

——. 1981b. "The Social History of Psychiatry in the Victorian Era." In *Madhouses, Mad-doctors, and Madmen: The Social History of Psychiatry in the Victorian Era,* edited by Andrew Scull.

Skultans, Vieda. 1975. *Madness and Morals: Ideas on Insanity in the Nineteenth Century.* London: Routledge and Kegan Paul.

——. 1979. *English Madness: Ideas on Insanity, 1580–1890.* London: Routledge & Kegan Paul.

Smith, Richard J. 1983. *China's Cultural Heritage: The Ch'ing Dynasty, 1644–1912.* Boulder, Colo.: Westview Press.

Smith, Roger. 1981a. "The Boundary Between Insanity and Criminal Responsibility in Nineteenth-Century England." In *Madhouses, Mad-doctors, and Madmen: The Social History of Psychiatry in the Victorian Era,* edited by Andrew Scull.

——. 1981b. *Trial by Medicine: Insanity and Responsibility in Victorian Trials.* Edinburgh: Edinburgh University Press.

Spence, Jonathan D. 1966. *Ts'ao Yin and the K'ang-hsi Emperor: Bondservant and Master.* New Haven: Yale University Press.

————. 1974. *Emperor of China: Self-portrait of K'ang-hsi.* New York: Vintage Books.

————. 1975. "Opium Smoking in Ch'ing China." In *Conflict and Control in Late Imperial China,* edited by Frederic Wakeman, Jr., and Carol Grant.

————. 1984. *The Death of Woman Wang.* New York: Penguin Books.

Sprenkel, Sybille van der. 1977. *Legal Institutions in Manchu China: A Sociological Analysis.* London: Athlone Press.

Staunton, George T. 1810. *Ta Tsing Leu Lee: Being the Fundamental Laws, and a Selection from the Supplementary Statutes, of the Penal Code of China.* London: Cadell and Davies.

Struve, Lynn. 1984. *The Southern Ming, 1644–1662.* New Haven: Yale University Press.

Sweeten, Alan R. 1976. "The Ti-Pao's Role in Local Government as Seen in Fukien Christian 'Cases', 1863–1869." *Ch'ing-shih wen-t'i* 3, no. 6:421–37.

Tseng, Wen-Shing. 1973. "The Development of Psychiatric Concepts in Traditional Chinese Medicine." *Archives of General Psychiatry.* 29:569–75.

Unschuld, Paul U. 1979. *Medical Ethics in Imperial China: A Study in Historical Anthropology.* Berkeley: University of California Press.

————. 1985. *Medicine in China: A History of Ideas.* Berkeley: University of California Press.

Valk, M. H. van der. 1948. "Dr. Karl Bünger, Quellen zur Rechtsgeschichte der T'ang-Zeit." *T'oung Pao.* 38:339–43.

Veith, Ilza. 1963. "The Supernatural in Far Eastern Concepts of Mental Disease." *Bulletin of the History of Medicine.* 37:139–155.

Wakeman, Frederic, Jr. 1985. *The Great Enterprise: The Manchu Reconstruction of Imperial Order in Seventeenth-Century China.* Berkeley: University of California Press.

Wakeman, Frederic, Jr., and Carol Grant, eds. 1970. *Conflict and Control in Late Imperial China.* Berkeley: University of California Press.

Walker, Nigel. 1967. *Crime and Insanity in England.* Vol. 1, Edinburgh: Edinburgh University Press.

Walton, John. 1981. "The Treatment of Pauper Lunatics in Victorian England: The Case of Lancester Asylum, 1816–1870." In *Madhouses, Mad-doctors, and Madmen: The Social History of Psychiatry in the Victorian Era,* edited by Andrew T. Scull.

Watt, John. 1972. *The District Magistrate in Late Imperial China.* Cambridge, Mass.: Harvard University Press.

Wu, Silas. 1970. *Communication and Imperial Control in China: Evolution of the Palace Memorial System.* Cambridge, Mass.: Harvard University Press.

Zelin, Madeleine, 1984. *The Magistrate's Tael: Rationalizing Fiscal Reform in Eighteenth-Century Ch'ing China.* Berkeley: University of California Press.

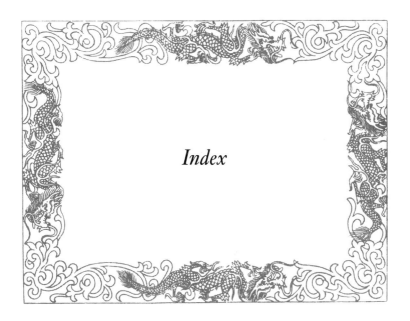

Index

Burial compensation, for family victim: 98

Canon of Filial Piety: as a political instrument, 17; *see also*, Xiaojing
Capital offenses, arbitration and review of: 20
Chastity, and statute of 1646: 15–16, *see* Women
chunyu, defined: 86
Clan: organization and control of, 76–78; elders, 66–68, 155
Clear-the-prisons edict, and the insane: 122
Clemency: for inadvertent offenders, 83, 100, 104, 118, 164; for the insane, 97, 164; for women, 138; by the emperor, 143; principle of, 147; petitioning for, 156
Climatic influences: 37; see also *wuyun liuqi*
Coherency, as proof of sanity: 105–6
Community drinking ceremony, as indoctrination: 12, 23, 167–68
Commutation: for hardened criminals, 157; for women, 162; requests for, 163
Competency, substatute of 1852: 106
Concealment, principle of: 70
Confinement, conditions of: 67
Confucianism: and humanity, 8; as state doctrine, 15–16; offenses against, 18; and propriety, 67; and Three Bonds, 94, 135; and the classics, 95; and filial piety, 96; and physicians, 166–67; and reform, 170
Confucianization of law: during Han, 15–16; to promote morality, 18; to a sanctified status, 22
Constables: and custody of the insane, 66; and recovery of insane, 67–68; and thieves, 69; registration of insane, 78; *see also* dibao
Cosmic correspondence, theory of: 18
Cosmic harmony: 15, 18–19
Crime: in Sichuan, 64–65; and the insane, 69, 74, 79; of husband-beating, 135–36; of wife-beating, 136–37
Criminal insanity: treatment of, 101; in 1776, 116–17
Criminals: control of, 75–77; and

criminal intent, 79, 83; claiming madness, 97; bonded statements, 155; mothers of, 155; petitioning for release, 157–58

Dai Sigong, Song-Yuan master: 45
Daoguang emperor: and parricide, 94–95; and amnesty, 123
Daoists: as healers, 28; using charms and incantations, 36; fasting for sinners, 52
Death penalty: executed by governor, 95; in Qing Code, 98; for insane murderers, 104, 106, 116, 123; by decapitation, 105; and amnesty, 123; and women, 138
Decapitation: for crimes of sudden insanity, 14; in Qing Code, 17, 98; for treason, 94; for multiple murder, 117
Deserving of Death, proviso for insane murderers: 115–16
dian: defined, 33; symptoms of, 34, 38; pathology of, 50
diankuang, in Qing encyclopedia: 33, 35
dibao: defined, 14; and social control, 23
Diminished responsibility: doctrine of, 86; use of, 118
Disease: in Chinese medicine, 28; diagnoses and observation, 34; causes of, 45
District Magistrates: and mandatory registration and confinement, 64, 66
Divine Retribution: as cause of madness, 79; *see also* Madness
Dong Zhongshu: on concept of *sangang*, 15; on theory of cosmic harmony, 18–19
dousha, defined: 97

Eight Trigrams Rebellion, of 1813: 95
Emotions: in madness, 28, 40; treatment of, 41
Emperor: as arbiter of justice, 20; intervention of, 140
Energy: routes of, 33–34; excess of, 50
England: treatment of madness, 51, 170; asylums, 60–61; insane offenders, 68; church and state, 69; homeless, 69; Hadfield case, 100–101; almshouses, 168; and Age of Reform, 169; psychiatry, 169